196710

THE MATURE YEARS:

A GERIATRIC OCCUPATIONAL THERAPY TEXT

Sandra Cutler Lewis, MFA, OTR

*Geriatric Supervisor for the
Department of Occupational Therapy
(Norristown State Hospital)*

*Occupational Therapy Consultant
to Long Term Care Service
(Norristown State Hospital)*

Cover photograph by Serena Nanda

Table of Contents

PREFACE vii

1 Challenging Ageism: Defining
   Attitudes That Affect the Dynamic
   Treatment of the Elderly Client 1

2 Theories of Growth and Aging 7
   Defining the Terms 7
   The Developmental Approach 7
   Aging Theory and the Therapist's Role 16

3 Biological and Physical Changes in Aging 19
   Frame of Reference 19
   Biological Theories.................................. 20
   Physical and Biological Changes..................... 22
   The Therapist's Function 29

4 The Socioeconomic Aspects of Aging 31
   The Retirement Years................................ 31
   Legislation 35
   The Therapist's Role 40

5 Primary Diseases of the Elderly 41
   Functional Disorders................................ 41
   Organic Disorders 45
   Physical Dysfunction 48

6 Treatment Programs and Techniques............... 61
   Reality Orientation 61
   Attitude Therapy 63
   Remotivation 64
   Opportunities for Increased Learning................ 65
   The Life Review 67
   Physical Conditioning Programs 68
   Physical Rehabilitation and
      Restorative Techniques 72
   Development of Sensory and Learning Skills 80

Utilization of Community Resources.................... 91
Client Determined Approaches to Treatment........... 92
Processes to Achieve Improved
   Sensorimotor Integration............................ 93
Craft Modalities for the Older Client 95

7 Coping with Death and Dying.......................101
Life and Death — A Comparative View 101
The Dying Process 103
New Programs on Death and Dying................. 106

**8 The Occupational Therapist as Consultant
and Private Practitioner 109**
Standards and Requirements......................... 109
Consultancy and Private Practice Settings 112
Interviews 113

9 Community Occupational Therapy Programs 121
Community-Oriented Programs 121
Home Health Care Agencies 126
Interviews 128

**10 Designing and Promoting Educational
and Informative Experiences.......................133**
Committee Structure and Responsibilities 133
Content... 134
Evaluations and Assessments....................... 134
Developing Community Information
   Exchange Projects 155

**11 Challenges for the Future —
Developing a Positive Therapeutic Model 159**
Myths About Aging.................................. 159
Elders Changing the Image 160
Stereotypes Concerning Occupational Therapy 162
The Promise of Tomorrow........................... 163

REFERENCES 165

BIBLIOGRAPHY 173

INDEX 175

Preface

The purpose of this book is to provide both a theoretical discussion of and a practical guide to geriatric occupational therapy. Included within this concept is an examination of the needs of the elderly as well as a compilation of practical therapeutic techniques and methods that are currently available to the geriatric specialist.

Particular acknowledgement is due Doris C. Kaplan, Director of the Occupational Therapy Department at Norristown State Hospital, who first suggested that I become involved in this type of project and whose thoughtful criticism and suggestions of the original manuscript have been essential in making this project a reality.

Special thanks are extended to Ginny Alpaugh, Evelyn Dietrich, RoseMarie Destra and Valerie Root for their time and effort in preparing the manuscript.

To the geriatric occupational therapy staff at the Norristown State Hospital—Stephanie Battjer, Dale Bassman-Ellenberg, Elizabeth Garrison, Kurt Hoff, Jeanette Liddle, John Livers, Susie Jackson, Marcie McGill, Jane Paire, Mary Shropshire, Laura Stravinskas, Barbara Valentine, and Wilma Wiener (Director of Education and Training of Occupational Therapy at Norristown State Hospital)—I would like to express my sincere appreciation for their sensitive approach to geriatrics and their support of me.

Finally, and most important, I would like to express my deep appreciation and love to Paul, Ethan, Judy, and Sharon Lewis who have been so very supportive and patient during these past months.

1

Challenging Ageism—

Defining Attitudes That Affect The Dynamic Treatment of The Elderly Client

At the onset of any discussion concerning geriatrics belongs an evaluation of current attitudes towards older citizens. Perhaps the greatest handicap that the elderly face is age prejudice. Few people would like to admit that they dislike elderly persons solely because they have lived a long time. Yet, our society fosters this very concept. Before therapists can assume a posture of helping professionals, it is necessary to carefully examine individual and societal attitudes so that these prejudices may be weeded out.

Where do negative attitudes towards aging arise? In *Aging and Mental Health: Positive Psychological Approaches*, ageism is defined as a "Systematic stereotyping of and discrimination against people simply because they are old."[1] The fear and dislike of growing old did not have its birth in our fast-paced twentieth century. Indeed, it was the ancient Greeks who idealized youth as beautiful. Love itself was personified as robust and young. Through the years the fear of aging has long been a part of human consciousness. The elixir of life and the fountain of youth of historical fame are but two examples of man's quest for eternal youth.

Elizabethan England was no exception to man's dread of the aging process. In William Shakespeare's *As You Like It*, Jacques describes the seven stages of man from infancy to old age. The closing lines..."Last scene of all, that ends this strange eventful history is second childishness and mere oblivion, sans teeth, sans eyes, sans taste, sans everything"[2] perpetuate the concept that the aged are primarily senile and helpless.

Therefore, we cannot say that it is only this century in which man has become critical of his aging brothers and sisters. However,

1

certain changes wrought by the full development of the Industrial Revolution and the Machine Age (for example, forced retirement) have only added a deeper message to Shakespeare's immortal lines. Formerly a person could work at his trade or profession within the community until he felt it was time to reduce his own work load. However, with today's mandatory retirement, many people experience a loss of identity at a premature age. In most instances, at 65, age segregation becomes enforced. The term *senior citizen* has become a familiar form of age labeling in our society.

Let us now examine contemporary literary comment. These reveal how our society perceives aging today.

Sharon Curtin spent many months traveling across the United States in quest of understanding what it is like to be old in today's America. In her brief statement..."We dote on youth. We shelve the old, and what does this say about how we view the whole of life?"...she gives us pause to think about our priorities concerning life's values.[3] Today there is indeed more than a generation gap. In our mobile society a true separation of the ages has evolved.

The Simon and Garfunkle *Bookend's* album, written when they were in their twenties, testifies to the significance of the separation and loneliness of the older person as viewed by the younger person.

Can you imagine us
Years from today,
Sharing a park bench quietly?
How terribly strange
To be seventy.
Old friends,
Memory brushes the same years.
Silently sharing the same fear...   Song 6 "Old Friends"

Time it was,
And what a time it was,
It was....
A time of innocence,
A time of confidences.
Long ago ...it must be ...
I have a photograph.
Preserve your memories,
They're all that's left you.   Song 7 "Bookends Theme"*

*Simon P, Garfunkel A: Bookends. New York, Charing Cross Music, 1968.

Television, one of this century's major mass communicators, has also played its role as an interpretor of the country's pulse. In the early days of television Edward Albee wrote a brief but poignant play, *The Sandbox.* These lines belong to Grandma:

> ...Honestly! What a way to treat an old woman! Drag her out of the house ... stick her in a car ... bring her in a pile of sand ...and leave her here to set. I'm eighty-six years old! I was married when I was thirty...I'm a feeble old woman... How do you expect anybody to hear me over the peep! peep!...There's no respect around here...
>
> They took me off the farm... which was real decent of them... and they moved me into the big town house with them... fixed a nice place for me under the stove... gave me a blanket... and my own dish... my very own dish! So what have I got to complain about! Nothing, of course I'm not complaining.[4]

The "Wall Street Journal," the very heartbeat of the business world, had this to report concerning a chronicled story of the plight of thousands of elderly persons in Los Angeles. Entitled "To be Old and Poor is to be Alone, Afraid, Ill-fed and Unknown," the article reported that... "many of the aged poor are depressed to the point of mental imbalance. The people who live near McArthur Park seem to have suffered sudden losses over a relatively short time span, viz loss of feelings or usefulness, etc. For many this is more than they can take." The article goes on to describe how some "eat dog food (they can get two meals out of a can). Where else can they get so much protein for so little money?"† When one thinks of the amount of advertising that is spent daily on feeding Fido or Tabby, it seems astonishing that the elderly poor's plight is not advertised with the same momentum.

Colloquial use of language often gives clues as to how the society views itself. Commonly used derogatory expressions such as "that old crab," "there's no fool like an old fool," "over the hill," "old fogy," and "old crock" are reminders that negative attitudes towards aging are ingrained patterns within the structure of our society. However, for the young, messages of endearment seem to prevail. For instance, the familiar lines of an old song "Mighty Like a Rose"— "Sweetest little fella, everybody knows"—lets one know that a young born baby is like heaven itself. Compare this to another old favorite like "The Old Gray Mare,"—"she ain't what she used to be,"

†*To be old and poor is to be alone, afraid, ill-fed and unknown.* Wall Street Journal, *November 15, 1972.*

and one can quickly surmise that it is normal to expect loss of vitality and ability as one ages.

The physical signs of aging—gray hair, wrinkled skin, arthritic hands, and shrunken frame—are not thought of by our society as beautiful. Like their ancient Greek counterparts, it is the youthful model that beckons us to believe that to be desirable, one must be young (or look young). Many cosmetic firms spend millions developing rinses and dyes that will hide "that tell-tale gray." Is it any wonder then that people within the health professions also feel this separation and noninterest for working with the elderly? Perhaps it is the fear of aging itself that prevents so many people from truly desiring to be involved with the health care of elderly persons.

In a recent interview for the *APA Monitor,* Dr. Butler, the first Director of The National Institute of Aging, answered the following questions with candor and concern.

Monitor: What role have the mental health professions played? What have they done to alleviate the mental and emotional problems associated with growing old?

Butler: Unfortunately, very little. They share society's ambivalence and negativism toward the old, but it's disguised in professional trappings. Their disinterest in the aged, combined with the often discrimination on the part of agencies and institutions, means that for most old people mental health services are unobtainable. Nursing homes, for example, rarely provide any form of psychiatric care, even though some 50 percent of their patients suffer from psychological problems and mental impairment. Those who are pushed out of mental institutions into boarding homes and other cheap living quarters have no follow-up mental health care: community mental health centers, for their part, see only a tiny portion of older persons. And private mental health services are simply too costly.[5]

Occupational therapists are no exception to this general attitude towards the elderly that is shared by their fellow health practitioners. In her article, "Occupational Therapy and the Aged," Jones reveals that "Many therapists see Gerontology as an unrewarding

4

and frustrating area of practice."[6] Some of the actual statements by therapists regarding attitudes towards gerontological clients include:

We are fighting a losing battle... There is little future in working with the elderly. They will only deteriorate more and die.

The progress and pace are too slow.

It is difficult to achieve positive and lasting results.

Even if the most advanced treatment techniques are applied, they will be meaningless if the client receives a negative message from his therapist.

At the turn of this century, 3.1% of the total population of the United States was over 65. Today 10% of the total population is over 65. By the year 2000 it is estimated that more then 32 million Americans will be over 65. When compared to previous generations, more persons of generally poorer mental and physical resources are now reaching old age.[7]

As the elderly population of the United States continues to grow, so too will the need for well-trained, competent geriatric specialists. At no time in the history of occupational therapy has the need for challenging and purposeful geriatric treatment programs been in greater demand.

2

Theories of Growth and Aging

Defining the Terms

Before one studies theories of growth and aging, the various aspects of the aging process should be clarified. Senescence involves the biological, psychological, and sociological changes that an individual experiences during different periods of his/her life. Although certain developmental characteristics occur at different times during the life cycle, each person ages at his own pace. The several components of aging include:

1) *Biological aging*—These are changes of the various biological and physiological processes that occur during the passage of time.

2) *Chronological aging*—The birth date is used to define an individual's age.

3) *Psychological aging*—These are changes in sensory functioning, perception, memory, learning, intelligence, and dynamics of personality that occur at various stages within the individual's life span.

4) *Sociological aging*—This includes the changing of roles, function, and status of the individual within the social system (ie, family, economics, governmental, recreational, religious affiliations, educational and medical).[1]

The theories in the remainder of this chapter represent a broad spectrum of thoughts concerning human development and aging.

The Developmental Approach

There are many theories concerning the aging process. Certainly, aging starts at the moment of conception and continues during the life span of the individual. The quality of human development as well as appropriate growth patterns are important components of developmental theory. These aspects of human growth are also important to geriatric practitioners because they help to identify the functioning level of the individual client.

The theories of Jean Piaget (cognitive development), Erik H. Erikson (psychosocial development), Lawrence Kohlberg (moral development), and Abraham H. Maslow (growth motivation) discuss developmental stages that are vital to one's maturation process.

Piaget's Theory

Jean Piaget's general theory of cognitive development is founded on two biological attributes—*organization* (tendency for living organisms to integrate processes into cohesive systems) and *adaptation* (the instinctive tendency of an organism to interact with his environment by means of assimilation and accommodation). The schema, an action sequence composed of organized sensori-motor responses, is a basic building block of his theory. An example of an inherited schema is the sucking pattern of a baby.[2]

Piaget's earliest theories deal with speech patterns of the young child. He postulates that the communication skills of the preschooler are "egocentric." The child rarely attempts to exchange thoughts with others. As the child grows older his speech becomes more socialized and he is able to consider another person's ideas.[3]

According to Piaget's theory there are five different developmental phases. Maturity encompasses the total integration of these stages. Some of the major characteristics of each phase are reviewed on pages 9-10.

Erikson's Theory

Cognitive development is but one of many aspects of human functioning. Psychosocial development offers another area of growth. Erik H. Erikson's work in this field details a series of eight phases or "ages" that he believes are essential to attain human maturity.

In each of these ages the individual struggles with two conflicting approaches or crisis situations. Erikson uses the word *versus* to demonstrate these polar differences. At each crisis phase the individual has options of positive or negative behaviors. The development of the individual occurs when he is biologically,

Chronological Order	Cognitive Modality	Characteristics
Birth to 2 yrs	Sensorimotor	*The Sensorimotor Phase* During this time the infant's earliest movements are primitive reflexes. Most learning occurs through the senses and by manipulation. Behavior during this phase can be categorized as "autistic." By age two the first internalization of schemata and the use of deductive thought may be utilized to solve problems. There are a total of six separate stages within the sensorimotor phase.
2 to 4 yrs	Preoperational	*The Preconceptual Phase* In the preconceptual phase the individual's thinking becomes more egocentric in approach. Play that emphasizes the why and how becomes the major tool for adaption. Symbolic play, simple language, and repetition are the mechanisms that are used. During this time the child is able to classify and compare items by a single attribute (for example, color or size).

4 to 7 yrs	Preoperational	*The Intuitive Phase*
		In this phase the individual truly begins to use words to express his ideas. The generalization of symbols as images becomes a major portion of the cognitive process. There is a gradual awareness of the conservation of mass, weight, and volume.
7 to 11 yrs	Concrete Operations	*The Concrete Operational Phase*
		This phase represents the utilization of logical thought. At this point the individual can organize objects into a series and is able to reverse operations (ie, addition and subtraction, multiplication and division). Communication and play are now used as a means of understanding the social and physical world. During this time the individual begins to gain a sense of autonomy.
11 to 14 yrs and ongoing	Formal Operations	*Formal Operations Phase*
		The concept of relativity, reason by hypothesis, and the use of implication begins to emerge. The individual is now able to understand abstract thought.[4]

psychologically, and socially prepared and able to move into the next phase. Erikson also uses the term *basic virtue* to represent realization of those values that he considers give meaning and spirit to human existence. Thus, each phase has its corresponding basic virtue. In regard to the first six ages, Erikson relates his developmental approach to Freudian psychosexual theory. The following represents a brief explanation of these eight ages or phases.

Chronological Order	Basic Virtue	Characteristic Ages (Phases)
Infancy	Hope	*Age I: Basic Trust vs Basic Mistrust*
		It is at this time that the infant learns to acquire a sense of trust by means of feeling physically well and by experiencing a minimal amount of anxiety. Behavior during this phase is egocentric.
Early Childhood	Will Power	*Age II: Autonomy and Pride vs Same and Doubt*
		During this time the individual begins to see boundaries between himself and his parents. Elimination and interest in the erotic areas of the body are of prime concern to the child, and he increasingly begins to assume a greater control of his body (regulation of the self vs regulation by others).

Play Age	Purpose	*Age III: Initiative vs Guilt*
		This is a period when the individual is expanding his language and mobility skills. Sexual identification also commences at this time. During this period the *id, ego,* and *superego* begin to find a mutual balance which leads to the fuller development of the personality.
School Age	Competence	*Age IV: Industry vs Inferiority*
		In this phase the individual develops his ability to win recognition by producing things. It is a time for systematic instruction. The child begins, then, to rely increasingly upon social institutions (schools, clubs, organizations).
Adolescence	Fidelity	*Age V: Identity vs Role Confusion*
		The individual physically matures into adulthood. He is constantly re-evaluating himself and his "new" body. Desire for sexual fulfillment begins to have more importance. According to Erikson, adolescence is a

		period of the moratorium, or delay between the child's world and the full responsibilities of the adult world.
Younger Adult	Love	*Age VI: Intimacy vs Isolation* The individual has the opportunity of becoming a full member of the society—enjoying both the responsibility (work world) and the liberty that is involved in adulthood. Ego-identity manifests itself during this period. This is usually the time that one acquires a mate and assumes mutual responsibilities that are involved (ie, regulate appropriate cycles of work, recreation, and procreation) with the given partner.
Adulthood	Care	*Age VII: Generativity vs Stagnation* During this phase the individual has the opportunity to guide the next generation. It is possible to achieve a sense of having contributed to mankind's future at this time.

Maturity	Wisdom	Age VIII: Ego Integrity vs Despair
		A spiritual sense pervades this final phase. It can be a time of fulfillment, acceptance, and respect for one's life style and life cycle.[5]

Kohlberg's Theory

The moral developmental theory of Lawrence Kohlberg represents another growth area of human functioning. According to Kohlberg there are six structured stages of development and a speculative seventh stage that reaches beyond the other stages to attain a humanistic perspective. The following are major characteristics of each stage.

Morality Level	Characteristic Stages
Preconventional	*Stage I: Punishment and Obedience* During this stage it is the physical consequence (ie, punishment, reward) that determines the value of an action. *Stage II: Instrumental Relativist* In this stage reciprocity becomes a major method of determining the value of an action (ie, "if you'll do this for me I'll do that for you").
Conventional	*Stage III: Interpersonal Concordance* Behavior is frequently judged by "intent." Approved behavior (often labeled as "good or nice") is determined by one's willingness to help others. There is conformity to stereotyped images.

Stage IV: Law and Order

Approved behavior is based upon one's willingness to respond to duty and respect for authority.

Post Conventional

Stage V: Social Contract Legalistic Approach

Approved action is based upon individual rights, with standards agreed upon by the society. However, these are not rigid but rather can be thought of in terms of free agreement and contract (with room for amending).

Stage VI: Universal Ethical Principle

"Right" action is determined by decisions of individual conscience as related to universal ethical principles (for example, "The Golden Rule").

Possible Stage VII: The Ontological-Religious Approach

This stage is still being defined by Kohlberg. It involves the contemplative experience and assumes an identification with the cosmic (infinite) perspective.[6]

Maslow's Theory

Another theoretician, Abraham H. Maslow, believed that mature human growth was dependent upon "need gratification or growth maturation." His theory is built upon the assumption that human beings fulfill their needs by a positive striving to grow. Maslow suggested a hierarchy of seven needs that commence with the most basic needs. As each lower need fulfills itself (by being appropriately and sufficiently gratified), the individual is able to move to the next need level. These hierarchical levels consist of the following needs: physiological needs, safety needs, belonging and love needs, esteem

15

needs, the need for self-actualization, the need to know and understand, and aesthetic needs.[6]

Opposing Theories of the Aging Process

Besides a developmental point of view of aging, there also exists two theories, *disengagement* and *active,* that are concerned with the way in which the individual and society views his/her own aging process.

According to Cumming and Henry, it is almost inevitable that as an individual ages and his personal resources decline, his interest in the social systems that he belongs to will also decrease. This withdrawal or disengagement can be seen by a decline in the number of people that an individual interacts with, the qualitative changes in patterns of interaction, and personality changes that result in decreased involvement.[7] This disengagement process helps the individual prepare for his eventual death.

Directly opposed to the disengagement theory is the *activity* theory. The majority of geriatric practitioners and theorists are proponents of this theory. Even though an individual may recognize his increasing limitations as he ages, old age may still be regarded as a time of fulfillment and as much activity as is possible. It can be a period when the wisdom of years may be harvested and utilized by the society. Like many other fellow professionals that support the activity viewpoint, Theodore Lidz believes that those people who continue to be involved in some form of productive activity remain alert for a longer period of time than those who are less active.[8]

Havighurst, Neugarten, and Tobin's findings pose yet another approach to the theories of aging. They regard an individual's personality as the cornerstone in predicting patterns of aging (social role activity and life satisfaction). Accordingly, as an individual grows older (if his personality remains integrated) there is an increasing consistency of that personality. For example, values that an individual has always felt positively about will become more cherished as he ages.[9]

Aging Theory and the Therapist's Role

The therapist's knowledge of a variety of aging theories facilitates his ability to comprehend more fully his client's behavior and capabilities. It is always important to present treatment programs that are responsive to the individual client's needs. Some examples of patient behaviors and how they relate to developmental theory follow.

The older person who is disoriented or who no longer can control his bodily functions experiences a sense of a loss of self. For instance, the incontinent person must cope with the frustration of feeling like a child as he is unable to regulate himself. Consider Erikson's *Age II—Autonomy vs. Shame and Doubt* as a comparison. Although some of the client's behavior may at times be reminiscent of a child's, he should not be treated as if he were a child. It should be remembered that this is a person who has experienced life, and that this chronological maturity deserves the respect of all staff members.

In the same vein, the older individual who is assessed as cognitively functioning at a 1½-year-old level (Piaget's sensorimotor phase) should be provided with treatment activities that reflect these findings (sensori-stimulatory). A treatment program that lies beyond the client's grasp can only result in disappointment and frustration for himself as well as the therapist.

The mentally alert older person, operating at a physically minimal level, represents yet another example of the varying complexities of human functioning. It is the therapist's obligation to make use of all the resources of his client. The developmental theories mentioned in this chapter discuss the number of stages that are necessary to attain maturity. The older person's wisdom and life experiences are indeed great strengths and assets that the therapist should utilize.

Another factor in resident care that has a direct bearing upon developmental theory is the relationship between the client and the institution. Institutional life may force many older people to assume behavior similar to Kohlberg's *Stage 3—Interpersonal Concordance* (good girl/boy label). For example, when the staff is preparing a special event like a trip, it is usually the "good patient," quiet and cooperative, who is permitted to participate.

In respect to Maslow's theory, the institutionalized older client's physiological and safety needs are usually met. However, higher level needs such as belonging and love, esteem, and self-actualization are usually not fulfilled. In this regard, the therapist has a very important mission as he/she can provide treatment that encourages the gratification of these more mature needs. For example, providing the client with opportunities to reclaim old skills (ie, cooking, sewing, gardening) can provide fulfillment in esteem and self-actualization needs.

Whether a person's life style dictates a disengagement pattern or one of activity, it is the dignity of the individual and his right to choose that should help to determine his treatment program. The therapist can help him in his decision making process and assist him in his efforts to accomplish specific treatment goals.

3

Biological and Physical Changes in Aging

Frame of Reference

As one ages, certain biological and physical changes occur. According to Strehler there are four characteristics that are common to senescence.

1) *Universality*—This concept asserts that specific aging characteristics can be seen in all segments of the elderly population. For instance, if gray hair is to be classified as a true phenomenon of aging, it must be shown that as people grow older, all subjects will exhibit some amount of graying hair.

2) *Intrinsicality*—The varying effects of ultraviolet radiation on both the physical and chemical properties of skin protein in young and elderly persons illustrates this characteristic. These effects depend on the changing susceptability of the skin collagen to irradiation and are not directly attributable to the ultraviolet light.

3) *Progressiveness*—True aging phenomena develops at a gradual pace and is generally not reversible. The development of atheroma and the resultant repair process which is seen by the accumulation of fibrous plaques on the intimal surfaces of the major vessels can be identified as an example of progressiveness.

4) *Deleteriousness:* Currently, there exists much controversy regarding this final characteristic. Accordingly, degradative and deteriorating changes must occur when senescence begins.[1]

Basically, there are two types of aging: 1) *primary aging*—a time related sequence closely rooted in heredity that results in a decline of

19

the efficiency of various functions within the organism, and 2) *secondary aging*—a process associated with stress, trauma, and disease.

Biological Theories

Busse affirms that human beings are composed of three biological components: 1) cells capable of multiplying throughout the life span (ie, epithelial and white blood cells), 2) cells incapable of division (ie, brain neurons), and 3) interstitial material (noncellular). He also states that the following biological theories of aging are based in part on at least one of these three components.

1) *Exhaustion Theory*—This rather dated biological explanation of aging assumes that an organism contains a fixed amount of energy. When this energy storage is depleted, the individual dies.

2) *The Accumulation of Harmful Material Theory*—This theory identifies aging with the accumulation of deleterious substances. The formation of lipofuscin (brown pigment) that is found in brain neurons as well as other cells of older persons is believed to be an example of this concept.

3) *Intentional Biological Programming*—Senescence occurs by means of programmed changes that take place within the life cycle of an organism. A specific example would be the human erythrocyte (one of the red blood cells) which appears to be programmed to live 120 years. Most research supports the assumption that there is a definite correlation between the survival of the erythrocyte and the total life span of the human organism.

4) *Decline in the Doubling Capacity of Human Cells*— The decline of the doubling capabilities of human cells is believed to be the causative factor responsible for senescence.

5) *Mean Time Failure*—Leonard Heyflick gives much credence to this theory which states that the life time of an organism is directly related to the durability of its parts.

6) *Accumulation of Copying Errors*—Aging occurs when one's cells develop copying errors that become amplified and widespread. Death takes place when the metabolic efficiency is

reduced, and ultimately when the cells lose their capability for repair.

7) *Stochastic Theories*—These theories focus upon cell loss or mutation as the main cause of aging. Laboratory studies demonstrate that the exposure of an organism to repeated small doses of ionizing radiation or to a larger sublethal dose reduces the life span of that organism.

8) *Curtis' Composite Theory*—Howard J. Curtis postulates that one ages because of the accumulation of defectively functioning cells in organs that are composed of nondividing cells. Further, Curtis believes that as one ages, one becomes increasingly susceptible to degenerative diseases. He asserts that an individual may develop all of the degenerative diseases at different rates before he or she dies.

9) *DNA-RNA Error Theory*—This theory of cellular aging assumes that as one ages alterations occur within the structure of the deoxyribonucleic-acid (DNA) molecule. These errors are then transmitted to ribonucleic acid (RNA), the messenger, and they are finally transmitted to newly synthesized enzymes. These defective enzymes could then produce substrates within the cell. The normal metabolic process might be seriously impaired. Death may result when the supply of RNA becomes too low for cell functioning.

10) *Eversion Theory (Cross-linkage)*—Senescence occurs when the collagen molecule (the most abundant protein in the human organism) alters its structure and changes its characteristics—especially its elasticity. This loss of elasticity accelerates the aging process.

11) *Autoimmunity*—As one ages, there is an increased incidence of autoimmune disease. This theory suggests that the gradual increase of antibodies (detected in the plasma) may be responsible for a lifelong accumulative exposure to multiple immunochemical substances.

12) *Index of Cephalization*—This hypothesis proposes that the excess of brain weight in relation to its expected body weight bears a direct correlation to longevity.

13) *Genetic Determinants of Aging*—While there is no specific gene that can insure a long life span, there are certain genes that are responsible for defects that result in shortening one's life. It is possible to theorize that an overabundance of

these genes would be responsible for an accelerated aging pace.[2]

Other theorists have proposed: 1) the *Lipid* (fat) *Peroxidation Theory* which asserts that unstable lipid portions of the lipoprotein cell membranes are continuously undergoing spontaneous peroxidation due to cosmic ray bombardment. Antioxidants such as vitamin E or alpha-tocopheral are believed to retard the peroxidation process (and presumably aging); and 2) the failure of the hypothalamus to regulate normal body functioning and rhythms.[3]

As research continues in its quest for the answer to the fundamental reasons of senescence, new theories may replace or alter the old ones. With the increasing amount of sophisticated technology that is being introduced yearly into the scientific community, one can assume that at some future date humankind will be able to understand the mystery of the aging process.

Physical and Biological Changes

The remainder of this chapter will discuss aging in terms of the physical, the biological, and the functional changes that occur within the human organism. However, there is considerable controversy as to whether these changes are due to intrinsic aging, wear and tear, or the consequences of vascular impairment and other diseases.

Throughout this section, specific discussion will be focused upon changes in the following areas: 1) the various systems of the body (respiratory, skeletal, nervous, muscular, reproductive, cardiovascular, urinary, and gastrointestinal tracts), 2) the skin and subcutaneous tissues, and 3) the senses (visual, kinesthetic, auditory, gustatory, olfactory, and tactile).

Systems of the Body

The Respiratory System

The three major components of the respiratory system—ventilation (breathing), diffusion (exchange of oxygen and carbon dioxide between the lungs and blood), and pulmonary circulation—show loss of efficiency as one ages. Specifically, this impairment can be seen by five symptoms:

1) the decline of total lung capacity.
2) an increase in residual volume.
3) a reduction in vital capacity. Research, conducted with 20-year-old subjects as compared to 80-year-old subjects, indicated that the breathing capacity declined from 132 liters per minute (20-year-old) to 50 liters per minute (80-year-old).
4) the decrease in the resiliency of the lungs.
5) the increasing thickening of supporting membrane structures between the alveoli and the capillaries.[4]

The Skeletal System

Skeletal changes typical of the aging process (such as stooped posture, stiffened joints, and porous bone structure) result in a decrease of mobility, efficiency, and capability of the human organism. These changes in appearance and function are manifested as:

1) a reduction in height.
2) poor posture—these postural alterations (partially bent hips and knees, stooping back, and flexed neck) are primarily due to a progressive calcification and eventual ossification of the ligaments (in vertebral ligaments this condition is often referred to as lipping vertebral). This mineralization process usually involves the elastic fibers; the erosion and ossification of cartilaginous joint surfaces as well as degenerative changes of the synovium. This process leads to an increased stiffening of the joints. The fibrocartilaginous discs undergo atrophic changes as they become thinner. These changes are particularly responsible for an increasing curvature of the spine and the atrophy of the boney structure of the vertebral and intervertebral discs and ligaments. These conditions result in kyphoscoliosis (hunched back).
3) atrophy of the ribcage area—degenerative changes in the rib cartilages and in the ligaments and joints which join the rib cage to the sternum and vertebrae are one of the causes of respiratory impairment.
4) loss of teeth—changes in the temporalmandibular joints and loss of teeth may cause difficulty in speech and eating.
5) increase in bone porousness—as one ages, the bones become more porous, lighter, and lose a great deal of their elasticity. This process actually is a disease state (osteoporosis).[4]

The Nervous System

The nervous system, also, undergoes a great deal of change. Within the brain itself, many changes can be identified as 1) a progressive atrophy of the gyri (convolutions) and the widening and deepening of the sulci (spaces between the convolutions), 2) a loss of the bulk of brain substances and dilitation of the ventricles which contain cerebrospinal fluid, 3) the progressive loss of neurons (many of the neurons that remain acquire lipofuscin, and 4) a progressive increase of corpora amylacea (small sand-like bodies) within the brain substance.[4]

Other changes within the nervous system are 1) a reaction time increase due to the degeneration of the integrative system, 2) an atrophy in the medullary olives, 3) a decrease in the Purkinje cells of the cerebellum, 4) trunk instability, and 5) losses within the proprioceptive, kinesthetic, vestibular and visual mechanisms. These mechanisms contribute to a characteristic gait which is considered typical of elderly persons (shorter step length, higher cadence, wider walking base, and a longer time period spent in the support stage of the step rather than the swing stage). Because of the combination of the increased reaction time and postural instability there is a greater tendency to fall as one ages.[5]

The Muscular System

The muscular system is another area that demonstrates decline during aging. Muscle atrophy, hypotonia, and muscle weakness are due to such multiple causes as 1) the thinning of individual muscle fibers, 2) the loss of nerve terminals, and 3) the diminished rate of synthesis of acetylcholine. As these muscle fibers degenerate, there is an increase of fat (ie, by age 70, fat may compose one third of the total dry weight of the gastrocnemius and fibrous tissue). The muscle loses a great amount of its ability to expand and contract at will because of these changes.[5]

As a result of this muscular deterioration, other bodily functions are also affected. These consist of impairment of respiratory efficiency, impairment of efficient excretory functions, and decline in the ability to respond effectively in an emergency situation. (The muscle is a major site for glycogen storage. Atrophied muscles lead to a loss of glycogen stores. This loss then results in an increased loss of reserve sugar from which is derived the energy that is required for use in emergency functioning).[4]

The Reproductive System

The major female reproductive change that occurs is menopause, a discontinuance of menstruation and the ability to bear children. This usually takes place at approximately 45-50 years of age. After menopause, there often is a gradual steroid insufficiency. This can cause the vaginal walls to become thinner and many women experience an increase of vaginal itching. However, steroid replacement therapy can alleviate these menopausal symptoms. Menopause does not deny women a satisfying sex life. In fact, many women maintain pleasurable sexual activity well into their seventies and eighties.[3]

The male "change of life" is often referred to as the climacteric. Many researchers feel that much of male impotency is directly due to lack of self-confidence. Although it may take an older man a longer time to obtain an erection, sexual capability can usually continue for as many years as the individual consistently pursues sexual activity. Men in their sixties and seventies have been known to have fathered children. Sperm has been found in persons 90 years of age.[6]

The Cardiovascular System

Some of the structural changes that occur include 1) an increase in interstitial fibrous tissue, 2) an increase of lipofuscin in the muscle cells, 3) an increase in amyloidosis (excessive deposits of starch-like material), 4) an elongation of the arteries which become tortuous and calcify, and 5) a thickening of the supporting membranes (including capillaries).

All these structural alterations contribute to the following changes in functioning: 1) there is a definite decline in cardiac output at rest; 2) the heart loses some of its capacity for responding to extra work; 3) there is a progressive increase in the peripheral resistance to blood flow, and the systolic blood pressure increases.

The Urinary Tract

In urinary tract functioning the filtration rate in the kidney of 80-year-old persons is approximately 50% of that of individuals in their twenties. The renal blood flow is also about 50%. Polyuria (excessive urination) is common. Structural changes such as the hyalinization of the glomeruli (kidney filters) and interstitial fibrosis are believed to result in the atrophy of the collecting tubules.

The Gastrointestinal Tract

Intrinsic aging of the gastrointestinal tract produces 1) a decline in stomach gastric mobility, 2) a reduction in gastric volume, 3) a tendency towards achlorohydria (loss of digestive acid), 4) a reduction in quantity of digestive enzymes, 5) a diminished peristalsis (this may be a factor that causes constipation, a common complaint of older persons), and 6) atrophy of the mucosal lining. This is responsible for the impairment of absorption that many older persons experience.[4]

The Skin and Subcutaneous Tissues

Gray hair and wrinkles, characteristics most often associated with an elderly appearance, yield a stereotyped image of older people. These characteristics can become symbols that may alter an older person's self-perception. Some of the areas of the body that display changes in external appearance are as follows.

Skin

Wrinkles—Wrinkling is often attributed to decreased blood supply and changes in collagen and elastic fiber. This results in a loss of elasticity and resiliency of the skin. When the skin is stretched in the older person, the folds become more delineated as they return into place.

Discoloration—During the aging process, the skin undergoes atrophic processes. Consequently there are many pigmentary discolorations (brown, yellow). Red blotches on the skin are usually caused by changes in the blood vessels beneath the skin.

Seborrheic keratoses—These are wart growths that appear to be stuck on.

Fissures—There appears to be an increase of fissures about the mouth. This may be caused by atrophy of the epidermal layer.

Nails

Atrophy of nail tissues causes the nails to become more brittle and grow at a slower pace.

Hair

There is a loss of hair pigmentation which results in its graying or whitening. This is believed to be due to a decrease in enzyme activity.

Tongue and Gums

The tongue and gum areas undergo atrophic changes and become reddened. Gum shrinkage around the teeth may cause eating and maintenance problems.

Subcutaneous tissue

This layer of tissue acts in two ways: as an insulator which helps to keep body heat constant and as a cushion against trauma. When these tissues atrophy, it becomes difficult for an individual to regulate body temperature.

Sweat and Oil Glands

The sweat and oil glands atrophy and decrease in size and number. Because of this, older persons lose their ability to sweat, and consequently, the skin becomes very dry.[6]

The Senses

The senses (auditory, visual, tactile, olfactory, gustatory, and kinesthetic) are the mechanisms by which the human organism gathers information about his environment. It is the senses that help us discern the differences between pleasant, unpleasant, and dangerous experiences. Imagine how difficult it would be to detect fire without the benefit of this type of alerting system. One would be unable to hear the crackling sound of fire, to smell the smoke, to feel the heat, or to see the flames.

Hearing Loss

Handicapping hearing impairments increase as one ages. Within the United States, there are nearly three million older people (+65) who have hearing impairments; of this number, 63,000 are classified as being totally deaf.

There are basically two different kinds of hearing loss: *conductive* and *sensorineural*. In conductive hearing loss, the sound has difficulty reaching the cochlea. This results in a loss of perceived intensity. Louder speech permits the person to hear adequately. Consequently, hearing aids are helpful.

27

Sensorineural hearing loss is characteristic of the type of degeneration that takes place during the aging process. Specifically, there is damage to some of the nerve endings in the cochlea. As a result, the ear responds to sounds in an uneven manner. There is usually a loss of one's ability to respond to high frequency sounds (such as the following consonants—s, t, p, k, and f). However, the low frequency sounds (usually vowels) are more readily heard. This results in the loss of the ability to discriminate words in speech. Speech is heard as muffled droning sounds of low frequency tones. Background voices (usually low tones) frequently mask the vowel sounds that a person can hear. Thus, if a television or an air conditioner are on during a conversation, a person with this type of hearing loss will not be able to fully comprehend what is being said. Hearing aids merely make the confused sounds louder and therefore are contra-indicated.

There are other types of conditions that impede hearing functioning. One of these is tinnitus. This is a high pitch "ringing in the ears." Another is presbycusis. This is a combination of discriminatory hearing loss and the presence of recruitment (faint or moderate sounds cannot be heard but loud sounds can be perceived). Functionally, a characteristic of presbycusis is a gradual reduction in sensitivity to high frequency sounds. Starting at approximately age 40, this condition increases in severity as the individual ages.[7]

Visual Loss

Visual loss can cause a decrease in mobility, frightening visual impressions, and poor orientation. By age 65, approximately 50% of the population in the United States experiences a visual acuity of 20/70 or less. At 75 years of age, three out of five persons experience some degree of visual loss.

Presbyopia is a condition that is caused by the inability of the lens to accommodate to far, near, and distant vision. The size of the lens increases gradually so that by age 80, it is 50% larger than at age 20. Comparably, the size of the pupil decreases and less light is able to reach the retina. Glare and the loss of the ability to adapt to sudden changes of light intensity are the two major problems that older persons experience.

Other conditions such as cataracts (clouding of the lens)

and glaucoma (increased intraocular tension) are responsible for impaired vision.[8]

Gustatory and Olfactory Loss

After age 50, a person's ability to discriminate and perceive the four taste qualities (sweet, salt, sour, and bitter) diminishes. By age 60, most people have lost 50% of their buds. Recent research demonstrates that the taste buds at the front of the tongue (sweet and salt flavors) atrophy first. Consequently, many older people complain that their food often tastes bitter and sour.

Since it is estimated that two thirds of taste sensations depend upon the ability to smell, there is a great interrelationship between these two senses. Approximately 40% of persons over 80 experience a decline of olfactory functioning. Consequently, many older people are no longer able to fully enjoy food or to detect differences in odors (harmful, pleasant, unpleasant). These losses greatly impair one's ability to operate with ease within his society.[8]

Kinesthetic Loss

The ability to perceive changes in body position and body orientation in space decreases with age. The changes are due, in part, to neurological and neuromuscular dysfunction, decline in muscular tone and strength, and dysfunction or disturbance of body mechanisms (ie, the vestibular system). Some older persons experience nystagmus, a constant, involuntary, cyclical movement of the eyeball. This causes them to perceive the ground or floor as moving up and down. Often, the deficits that impede appropriate kinesthetic functioning compel the older person to compensate by changing his gait patterns (ie, a longer amount of time is spent in ground contact).[8]

Tactile Loss

As one ages, there is a gradual loss of the ability to perceive heat, cold, and feel touch sensations. The vibration sense of the extremities may also be lost.[4]

The Therapist's Function

Much of this chapter has dealt with the physical, biological, and

29

functional decline of the older person. Whatever the situation, it is the treatment of the "whole" person—not just an isolated body part—that should reign supreme.

Because so many areas of decline and dysfunction overlap from one to another, the therapist should be well acquainted with the complete spectrum of the aging process. For instance, if one is treating a confused, depressed older person, it is important to be aware that this person may also be experiencing a kinesthetic loss. If this is true, then appropriate self-help aids (ie, grab rails in the hall) and proprioceptive input should be considered as much a part of treatment as reality orientation and life review. Similarly, if the treatment of a 75-year-old client includes "development of ADL skills" (ie, learning to be more self-sufficient in the kitchen), it is good to note that certain olfactory and gustatory cues (such as being able to distinguish the aroma of different spices) may not be able to be utilized. Thus, with this knowledge the therapist can adapt treatment requirements (involving the use of large print labeling and color coding of the spice containers) to meet the needs of his client.

It is essential that the geriatric practitioner be aware of the consequences of decline that are associated with intrinsic aging. The therapist who comes armed with as much information as he can acquire is able to deal more competently in initiating and maintaining effective treatment programs than one who has kept his scope of knowledge to narrow confines.

4

The Socioeconomic Aspects of Aging

The Retirement Years

Since the advent of social security, initiated under Franklin D. Roosevelt's administration, age 65 has become the established cut-off point between the working world and the world of retirement. During these years one becomes more isolated as most of his/her former and familiar social supports (ie, the family, job status, income) begin to diminish. It takes enormous personal strength on the part of the older person to face the many losses that are interlaced within this life period.

Coping With Physical Loss

In the preceding chapter the physical changes that occur with aging were discussed. Not only is there physical decline but often disease accompanies these physical conditions. The older person must then learn to cope and adjust to these changes. More energy is needed and spent in the care and the maintenance of the body. Because of these types of concerns, whole new patterns of life need to be initiated. Examples of this can be seen in the older person who can no longer dine out because of gastrointestinal problems, or the person who can no longer drive an automobile because his visual acuity has declined.[1] A great deal of independence must be relinquished as one becomes increasingly dependent upon others to perform services that previously had been done by the individual. As the social world begins to diminish, separation from the community and loneliness often become an established consequence.

Adjusting To The Permanent Loss Of A Job

According to the theories of Friedman and Havighurst, work assumes the following five universal functions:

1) **Provides income**—Income is the substance from which the physical necessities and luxuries of life are obtained.

2) **Regulates life activity** (energy and time)—Work usually determines the hour that one rises; the time that one eats breakfast, lunch and dinner; the length of vacations and holidays; the types of clothing that one wears (for at least five days out of seven); and the workers residential area (which includes rural, urban, or suburban life style associations).

3) **Offers identification and status**—Often when a person is introduced to another the question, "What do you do?", is invariably asked. One is identified with the occupation that he pursues.

4) **Provides opportunities to associate with others**—During the work period one usually comes into contact with other individuals. Coffee breaks and lunch hours are often shared with coworkers.

5) **Makes available opportunities for a meaningful life experience**—This is especially true if one enjoys and takes pride in his work.[2]

If these are the attributes that work provides, the adjustment to these losses will present paramount changes in the individual's life patterns. New activities should seek to offer similar satisfactions that a worker had experienced during his years of employment.

Adjusting To Lower Income Levels

Retirement often means facing society on a fixed and lower income then one was accustomed to prior to separation from the work world. Savings of a lifetime may be spent quickly by prolonged illness. In the past 30 years we have been experiencing periods of great inflation. This too, unfortunately, aides in impoverishing many older citizens. Thus, the very needs and staples of life (food, clothing, and housing) can become luxuries.

Coping With Changing Roles

Old age is a time in which the American society does not readily assign clearly defined roles. In fact, it is a time for permanent disengagement from two firmly entrenched social structures—the nuclear family and the occupational system.[3] The older person actually loses a sense of whom he/she is when terminated from the work force. No longer a teacher, chemist, or active parent, his identity suddenly vanishes. He, therefore, becomes a person without a place.

In other parts of the world where respect and honor are accorded the elderly, it has been found that these older people rarely retire from the work world or their community. For instance, centurians from the South Altay and Caucasus areas chair many community functions (celebrations, weddings, and dinners). They are considered to be wise and have a special place in their society. It is not uncommon for people from these regions to live well beyond 100 years.[4]

Dealing With New Housing Needs

The repair, cleaning, and maintenance of a house that one has lived in for 25 years or more may become increasingly too burdensome. Moving away from lifetime memories and the decline of complete independence is another in a long series of losses that many older people experience. Some housing alternatives may be foster homes, retirement centers, smaller apartments, boarding homes, moving in with one's children, cooperative housing, or for the more physically impaired, a nursing home. Often certain adaptive devices (raised toilet seats, grab rails) need to be employed to encourage as much independence as possible.

Unfortunately, many residential halls and nursing homes still retain the custodial climate of their predecessors—the almshouse or the poor house. Most older people believe that these places are degrading. Some of their complaints of the traditional institutional model are that the institutions are custodial in nature; the residents are expected to play a passive role rather than one that reflects physical and mental activity; the individuality of the client is compromised for group conformity; the staff is impersonal and over-professional; and many of these institutions expand in size beyond the optimum level so that the per capita cost can be reduced.[2]

Coping With The Loss Of
Life Partners, Family, and Friends

The elderly spend tremendous amounts of emotional and physical energy that is directed to grieving and the resolving of grief. It is a time when the deaths of a spouse, brother, sister, or close friend may be steps apart from each other. For many it is the beginning of a solitary life and great change. The family residence may become unmanageable or unwanted by the remaining partner. Funeral arrangements, burial preparations, and the disposition of the spouse's personal effects are some of the emotional yet practical aspects that accompany the mourning process. For most women, who outnumber men by a three to one margin, it is unlikely that they will be able to find another partner.[5]

Society And The Elderly Look For New Solutions

Although this is a period of multiple losses for most older individuals, many elderly people are becoming more vocal in making society aware of their needs. The National Caucus for the Black Aged, the Gray Panthers, the Senior Action Alliance Centers, the American Association of Retired Persons, the National Council of Senior Citizens, and the Gray Bears are some examples of action groups which assume an advocate role for older people.

Magazines such as "Modern Maturity" and "Retirement Living" that focus on the needs of the older consumer are becoming more popular.

In recent years the federal government, also, has been taking an increasingly active role in providing funds for services and programming for older persons. The most significant legal action has been the passage of The Older Americans Act.

Legislation

The Older Americans Act

This act was first established on July 14, 1965 (Public Law 89-73) and has been amended by Public Law 90-42 (July 1, 1967), by Public Law 91-69 (September 17, 1969), and by Public Law 93-29 (May 3, 1973). The purpose of the latest amendments, known as *The Older Americans Comprehensive Service Amendments of 1973*, was to strengthen and improve the original Older Americans Act of 1965. There are now a total of ten titles.

Title I: Declaration of Objectives
The purpose of this title is to make available comprehensive social service programs to older Americans and to provide the opportunity for them to participate in the development of these programs.

Title II: Establishment of the Administration on Aging
The Administration on Aging, headed by the commissioner on aging, is placed within the Office of the Secretary of Health, Education and Welfare. It provides for the creation of a National Information and Resource Clearing House for the Aging. In addition, this title establishes a Federal Council on Aging.

Title III: Grants for State and Community Programs on Aging
The Administration on Aging is committed to work with state agencies on aging (sometimes referred to as the Area Agency on Aging) in developing state-wide plans for the delivery of social services to older citizens. Special grants may be given to projects involving housing needs, transportation needs, continuing education, preretirement information, services to the handicapped, and for demonstrations (available to public and private nonprofit agencies).

Title IV: Training and Research
Direct grants and contracts may be awarded to research and development projects in the field of aging. Funds are also available for the specialized training of employed persons or those persons preparing for employment in programs devoted to aging. There are also provisions for establishing and supporting multidisciplinary centers of gerontology.

Title V: Multipurpose Senior Centers

This section provides for the construction, acquisition, alteration, and renovation of multipurpose senior citizen centers. Included also are funds for mortgage insurance and grants for staffing these centers.

Title VI: National Older Americans Volunteer Program

Authorization is granted to establish the Foster Grandparents Program and other Older Americans Community Service Programs (transferred to the Action Agency in 1971). These are designed to involve older Americans in programs that benefit persons of all ages. Some examples include:

RSVP (Retired Senior Volunteer Program)—These are service volunteer programs in public and nonprofit institutions.

SCORE (Service Corps of Retired Executives)—Under this program retired businessmen advise novices in the field of business management.

VISTA (Volunteers in Service to America)—This program, designed for persons of all ages, provides community service projects for at least one or two years duration.

PEACE CORPS—Volunteers of all ages are involved in community programs in foreign countries for usually a two year tour of duty.

Title VII: Nutrition Programs

The purpose of this title is to promote greater coordination between nutrition programs and the social service programs that were provided in Title III (ie, meals on wheels, congregate meals served in senior centers, synagogues and churches).

Title VIII: Amendments to Other Acts

This section provides opportunities for older Americans to participate in programs of continuing education that are expanded by amending the following acts: Library Services and Construction Act, National Commission Libraries and Information Science Act, the Higher Education Act, and the Adult Education Act (ie, book mobiles, library services offered to bed-bound patrons).

Title IX: Community Service Employment for Older Americans

Community service jobs are provided for low income Americans 55 years of age and older in the following fields:

education, recreational services, social services, conservation, economic development, and environmental restoration. Most of the programs utilize the experiences of demonstration projects that are conducted by the Department of Labor under its Operation Mainstream Program. Some of these programs are Operation Green Thumb for men (conservation and landscape) and Operation Green Light for women (community service programs). Both of these programs are sponsored by the National Farmers Union. Other community service programs are the Senior Aids (sponsored by the National Council on the Aging) and the Senior Community Service Aides (sponsored by the National Retired Teachers Association).

Title X: Middle Aged and Older Workers Training Act

The main objective of this title is to provide manpower training programs and other services to improve and increase job opportunities for the middle-aged and older citizen.

Other Federal Regulations, Acts, Laws, and Programs Affecting Older Persons

The mission of the law PL 93-296 is the creation of the National Institute of Aging. Its purpose is conducting and supporting social, biomedical, and behavioral aspects of training and research as related to the aging process, the diseases of the elderly, and other special problems of older Americans. There are two types of research programs. Intramural research is conducted in Baltimore at the National Institute on Aging which was formerly known as the Gerontology Research Center. Extramural research is administered by the Adult Development and Aging Branch. Included in this program is the development of many multidisciplinary centers for aging research.

The National Institute of Mental Health Grant Programs for Staff Development in Hospitals, a federally funded staff development program, is designed to improve the development of patient treatment within public mental health hospitals (including those within state hospital systems). The program includes inservice training for nonprofessionals and professionals. The content may include orientations, continuing educational courses, refresher programs, and special courses for teachers who conduct the training. Because of the large numbers of older patients within the state hospitals, this type of grant program can have a positive effect on the type of care that these elderly citizens receive.

Programs Supported by the Social Security Administration — Hospital/Medical Coverage

In the Hospital Insurance Program (included in Title XVIII: Medicare), hospital insurance services are offered to any person 65 years of age or older and to those entitled to social security/railroad retirement benefits (a dependent spouse 65 or over is also eligible for this coverage). In each benefit period the covered protection includes hospital inpatient care; posthospital extended care, and home health visits by nurses and other allied health workers from a participating home health agency. Physicians fees are not covered. These benefits, financed under social security, are based upon contributions (from workers, their employers, and self-employed persons) made during their working years. This portion of the contribution is held in a special Hospital Insurance Trust Fund.

The Supplementary Medical Insurance (included within Title XVIII: Medicare) is part of the social security program which helps to pay for physician's bills, outpatient hospital services, medical services and supplies, home health aide services, and rehabilitative outpatient health care services. This program, financed by voluntary supplemental extensions of Medicare's hospital insurance program, is not financed by payroll deductions.

Under the Medical Assistance Program (under Title XIX: Medicaid) grants are provided for individual states to administer programs that assist certain people:

1) public assistance recipients who are aged, blind, disabled, or dependent children.
2) those who are medically needy (but not public assistance recipients) and who represent the same group as mentioned in category one. These citizens may have sufficient income for daily needs but not enough finances to cover medical expenses.
3) any child below the age of 21 whose parents cannot afford medical care.

Possible Funding Sources for Geriatric Day Care Programs, Public Law 92-603 (under Title XVIII Part B and Title XIX of the Social Security Act), provides for the opportunity to implement geriatric day care programs.

Model Cities Funding: The National Council on the Aging (through Title IV, Part A of the Social Security Act of 1971 and Titles I and XVI of the 1972 Social Security Act) is responsible for funding special services in model cities.

Resources

Amendments and alterations to existing laws are constantly taking place. Information regarding current public health care programs and regulations may be obtained by writing to the *Federal Register,* the National Archives of the United States, Washington, D.C.

Another source that includes information regarding federal benefits and programs is the Printing Office of the Department of Health, Education and Welfare, Social Security Administration, Washington, D.C.

The federal government is not the only source of third party payments to medical services. Supplemental health insurance policies for older Americans is provided by Blue Cross/Blue Shield; National Council of Senior Citizens; American Association of Retired Persons; and many other commercial carriers.

White House Conferences on Aging

There have been two White House Conferences on Aging (1961—called by President Eisenhower, and 1971—called by President Nixon). Previously Harry S. Truman had called a National Conference on Aging in 1950.

The 1971 White House Conference on the Aging was attended by more than 3,000 people. Some of the many issues discussed were improving the transportation needs of the elderly, providing better housing for older persons, improving the medical delivery system, increasing nutrition programs, and improving the financial status of older people. One very significant aspect of the 1971 conference was that the elderly themselves were encouraged to testify and to participate in the development of future programming.[6]

Looking Towards the Future

Within the past 25 years, older Americans have become increasingly vocal about their needs. Legislation, conferences, and a variety of services from both the public and private sector have been established to combat and improve the multiple problems that older citizens face.

As the population of the United States grows older, new life patterns may begin to emerge. Some thoughts to consider might be extending the retirement age to a later period in one's life span, partial retirement, or a shorter work week. One can feel certain that as our population's needs shift, so too will the attitude within our society. Because an older person is in the unique position of being fully able to comprehend the total life cycle, this wisdom and life experience can be utilized to help guide society.

The Therapist's Role

The dynamics of aging should be well understood by therapists before they become practitioners. These dynamics not only reflect how the elderly feel about themselves but also what society expects of them.

Although most elders are experiencing physical decline, a lower standard of living, and emotional losses, the life experience and maturity of the older person should definitely be a contributing factor in determining methods of dealing with their problems. An understanding of these varying components should be the foundation for developing appropriate treatment plans.

Geriatric specialists should also be knowledgeable about the latest legislative programs that are offered to older persons. This will enable therapists to inform their clients of the services that are available and to have a more thorough understanding of current funding sources. With this information the geriatric practitioner can then become involved in initiating creative and meaningful treatment opportunities for their clients.

5

Primary Diseases of the Elderly

Statistics indicate that 86% of older persons have some form of chronic health problem.[1] It is not unusual for the elderly to experience two, three, or four diseases or areas of dysfunction simultaneously. Many of these chronic physical problems are accompanied by varying degrees of pain.

Mental (Psycho-Social) Dysfunction

During late life one is most likely to develop some form of mental illness, specifically a functional or organic brain disorder.[2] These two types of mental illness have very different origins. Functional disorders (which include such affective disorders as depression, paranoia, schizophrenia, neurosis, personality disorder, alcoholism, and drug dependence) appear to be emotionally based while organic disorders are firmly rooted in a physical foundation.[1]

Functional Disorders

Depression

The incidence of depressive illness tends to increase with advancing age. In fact, suicides account for 27.9 deaths per 100,000 population of people in the 75 to 85 year age bracket.[3]

Depression can manifest itself in many ways—self-reproaches; negative self-concepts; a specifically altered mood which shows itself in terms of apathy, loneliness, sadness; a retarded activity level; a definite loss of libido (expressed by insomnia and increased anorexia); and regressive and self-punitive wishes (such as desires to escape, hide, or die).[4]

With an older person, depression is complicated by several

41

external factors. First is the repeated experience of *loss*—a spouse or friend, a talent, a body part or function. A second factor is the relentless *attack* of nature (either physically or psychologically) on an aging body, causing discomfort, injury, and pain. Third is the frustrating *restraint* imposed on older life by various disorders (for example, the bed rest required by certain diseases, the restricted activity prescribed for heart patients, even the economic limitations imposed by a fixed income). The combined and repeated experience of these factors results in a constant state of *threat*, evoked at the smallest sign of an impending loss, attack, or restraint.[5]

It is often difficult to distinguish between depressive and organic states. However, the major types of depression which most affect older persons include mood disorders (both involutional melancholia and manic depressive psychoses), psychotic depressive reactions, and depressive neuroses.

Involutional melancholia (or involutional psychotic reaction) was originally associated with menopause but is now associated with aging in general. Onset of the disorder occurs during the ages of 40 to 50 in females and 50 to 65 in males. The depression characteristic of this disease can be manifested in guilt feelings, reduced self-regard, anxiety, insomnia, somatic preoccupation, agitation, and delusory ideas. It is not linked to a previous history of manic-depressive illness.

Manic-depressive psychoses are marked by periods of severe mood swings (elation to depression) which may occur as cyclic episodes of one mood alone or of both extremes.

Psychotic depressive reactions are severe symptoms of depression that can be attributed to a definable life experience (such as a serious loss or disappointment). In such a state, a person has only a tenuous grip on reality, and his ability to function may be greatly impaired.

Depressive neuroses (also termed depressive reactions or reactive depressions) are the most common neuroses of older persons, often initiated by loss of a loved one, disappointment, criticism, or threats (both imagined and real).[1]

Current research on depression is focusing more and more on the biochemical factors involved. Many typical depressive behaviors can be related to such specific biochemical changes as higher salt retention within the cells, production of larger amounts of cortisol (a hormone that comes into play during periods of body stress), heightened heart and respiration rate, clenched body musculature, and apparent disorganized hyperactivity of the central nervous system (causing nervous circuits to operate inefficiently).

Perhaps the most important recent findings concern the biogenic amines, substances that are released by the brain's nerve cells which appear to affect and alter moods. Some scientists now believe that a balance of norepinephrine (a biogenic amine credited with being a primary factor of arousal and alertness), serotonin (another amine believed to be associated with drowsiness), and perhaps other lesser known biogenic amines is essential to maintaining normal moods.

Other scientists believe that the enkephalins and endorphins (pain killers which occur naturally in the brain) may be more important than the biogenic amines in affecting mood.

In 1972 the MHPG (3-Methoxy-4-Hydroxyphenylglycol) compound, which derives from norepinephrine, was discovered in the urine and in the cerebrospinal fluid of human and animal subjects. Dr. Schildkraut, a professor of psychiatry at Harvard, believes that MHPG will prove clinically helpful both in determining the different types of depression and in predicting how well a patient will respond to different types of antidepressants.*

Nondepressive Functional Disorders

Besides the depressive disorders, there are a number of psychiatric illnesses which affect older persons: schizophrenia, paranoia, several types of neuroses and personality disorders, and psychophysiological disorders.

Schizophrenia, a disease marked by disturbances of thought, mood, and behavior, is characterized by hallucinations, poor contact with reality, delusions, diminished control of impulses, and inappropriate behavior and attitudes. The disease, as it affects the elderly, falls into two major types: *chronic* and *senile*. Chronic schizophrenia refers to a disease whose symptoms originated in adolescence. Persons with this type of schizophrenia have carried their behaviors and mental disturbances from adolescence into late life. Senile schizophrenia refers to the disease which develops only in late life; it is a rare disorder.

---

*Scarf M: From joy to depression: New insights into the chemistry of moods. The New York Times Magazine, April 24, 1977, pp 31-37.

43

Paranoid states are psychotic disorders manifested by a delusion, usually of a grandiose or persecutory nature. The delusion may cause disturbances in mood, behavior, and thinking although it does not impair intellectual functioning. Paranoia tends to occur when a person is suffering under an adverse condition such as blindness, deafness, isolation, or infection. It is believed that the isolation from human contact which occurs with hearing loss or blindness results in the misinterpretation of incoming stimuli.

Neuroses, while they may impair thinking and judgment, do not manifest as gross a distortion of reality or as profound a disorganization of personality as do the psychotic disorders (schizophrenia and paranoia). According to psychiatric theory, neuroses are the result of attempts to resolve unconscious emotional conflicts. Characterized by anxiety, neurotic conditions are very common in late life.

The neuroses that appear most frequently in old age include depressive neuroses (discussed on p. 42), hysterical neuroses (both dissociative and conversion types), obsessive-compulsive neuroses, phobic neuroses, and hypochondriacal neuroses.

With dissociative hysterical neurosis, the older person becomes extremely anxious to the point of personality disorganization. This state often results in amnesia, confusion, fatigue, and stupor. With conversion hysterical neurosis, a person manifests emotional conflict through physical symptoms; his autonomic nervous system is not involved.

A person suffering obsessive-compulsive neurosis repeats thoughts or actions, unable to discontinue the pattern.

Someone in a phobic state repeatedly exhibits an intense fear of something; this fear displaces some real feared object or event.

With hypochondriacal neurosis, a person is overconcerned with his own well-being. He may complain of various bodily ailments for which there is no actual physiological basis. These ailments serve his needs in a variety of ways: punishment for guilt, a method of controlling others, a symbol of his deterioration and age, a displacement of anxiety, a method of inhibiting undesired behavior, a means of reducing interpersonal contact, and a method by which he can identify with a deceased loved one who may have experienced similar symptoms. There is a great deal of overlap between hypochondriases and depression.

Personality disorders cover a whole group of old age disorders which are the result of personality defects developed over a lifetime. The following are examples of deeply ingrained maladaptive patterns of behavior often observed in older persons: schizoid, paranoid, inadequate obsessive-compulsive, cyclo-thymic, hysterical, explosive, asthenic-antisocial, and passive-aggressive.

In psychophysiological or psychosomatic disorders the physical symptoms are caused by emotional factors. However, there are definite differences between this disease state and conversion reactions or hypochondriases. Psychophysiological disorders involve the autonomic nervous system; they do not help to reduce anxiety. The symptoms are physiological rather than symbolic. Since actual structural change occurs, these disorders pose a definite somatic threat. The most common psychosomatic reactions of older persons are pruritus (of the ani and vulvae), psychogenic rheumatism, irritable colon, nocturia (frequent urination at night), cardiac neuroses, preoccupation with bowel habits, and hyperventilation syndromes.[1]

Organic Disorders

Fifteen percent of people in the 65 to 75 year age bracket and 25% of people 75 years and older have been diagnosed as "senile." Currently, most professionals refer to this mental state as "organic brain syndrome."†

Diagnostic Methods

The arrival of the CAT (computerized axial tomagram), a revolutionary new X-ray technique, has made possible a more definitive neurological diagnosis of this syndrome. Quick and painless, the CAT X-ray actually shows a shrunken brain.† Previous clinical diagnostic measures (such as the EEG, the static and dynamic brain scans, cerebral angiography, ultra-sound, pneumoencephalography, and cisternography) were time consuming,

---

†*Altman LK: Medicine — Senility is not always what it seems to be.* New York Times, *May 8, 1977, p 9e.*

sometimes painful, and not very accurate.

Other diagnostic evaluations and assessments, however, are helpful in determining the severity of the condition: they include the Mental Status Evaluation (S. Perlen and R.N. Butler), the Mental Status Questionnaire (R.L. Kahn, A.I. Goldfarb, M. Pollack, and A. Peck), the Short Portable Mental Status Questionnaire (E. Pfeiffer), Double Simultaneous Stimulations of the Hand and Face (A.I. Goldfarb), the Bender Visual-Motor Gestalt Test (Bender), and self-drawings.

Organic Brain Syndromes — Acute and Chronic

Organic brain syndromes are psychiatric disorders that reflect brain cell loss or impairment of brain tissue function. They fall into two basic types: *acute* (reversible) and *chronic* (irreversible).

There are five traditional signs which indicate organic brain dysfunction: impairment and disturbance of memory, impairment of intellectual functioning, impairment of orientation, impairment of judgment, and labile or shallow affect.[1] However, psychiatric, neurotic, and behavioral disorders may complicate the clinical picture of any organic brain dysfunction.

Acute brain syndrome may result from:

1. cerebral hypoxia, decreased oxygenation of the blood caused by anemia, pulmonary disease and similar factors;
2. increased cerebral oxygen requirement such as that found in thyrotoxicoses and febrile states;
3. insufficient supply of a necessary metabolic substance such as nicotinic acid and thiamine;
4. a disruption of cerebral metabolic processes (manifested in endocrine disorders, head trauma, toxic states, or fluid and electrolyte imbalance);
5. impaired cerebral blood supply (seen in cardiac disease, hypertensive encephalopathy, and decreased blood volume).[6]

One consistent characteristic of acute brain syndrome is that the pathology is reversible. Other symptoms of the disorder include a fluctuating level of awareness, hallucinations (particularly visual), disorientation, loss of remote and recent memory, restlessness, a dazed expression, aggressiveness, delusions of persecution, anxiety, and lack of cooperation.[1]

46

Chronic brain syndrome, diffuse brain damage with massive loss of cortical and limbic neurons, can be caused by a number of circumstances including:

1. episodic and recurrent blood loss (caused by infections with high fever, cardiac arrhythmia, anemic states, myocardial infarction, and blood pressure drops) which develops slowly and insidiously;
2. erosion of vulnerable areas of the brain which are poorly supplied by collateral blood vessels (leading to erosion of total mass of brain tissue);
3. occlusion of the arterioles (because of thromboses or emboli) which results in a critical loss of cerebral tissue;
4. cerebral degeneration of unknown origin (such as that manifested by presenile sclerosis) which can occur at any age.[6]

The emotionally laden term *senility* refers specifically to chronic brain syndrome. The primary characteristic of this syndrome is its irreversibility. Dr. R.N. Butler considers organic brain syndrome to be divided into two categories: *senile psychosis* (senile dementia/ senile brain disease) and *psychosis* associated with cerebral arteriosclerosis.[1] On the other hand, Dr. A.I. Goldfarb believes that organic brain syndrome should be classified as *uncomplicated* (irreversible cognitive impairment without any appreciable degree of thought, behavioral, or mood disorder) and *complicated* (irreversible cognitive impairment that is accompanied by disturbances of thought, content, behavior, or mood).[6]

Senile Psychosis

In senile psychosis there is a progressive decline in mental functioning associated with structural changes within the brain caused by atrophy and degeneration. Early features of senile psychosis include errors in judgment, decline in self-care habits, loosening of inhibitions, impairment of abstract thought, restlessness, depression, and anxiety. These symptoms are precursors of greater impairments.

Arteriosclerotic Psychosis

While senile psychosis shows a steady mental decline, arteriosclerotic psychosis is characterized by an uneven downward progression. This disorder is associated with the arteriosclerotic impairment of the cerebral blood vessels. Early symptoms include dizziness, headaches, and a decrease in vigor. Another important characteristic is erratic impairment of memory.

Presenile Dementia

Presenile dementia refers to a group of cortical brain diseases (Alzheimer's disease and Pick's disease are the most common) which clinically resemble the senile dementias seen in older persons. Presenile dementias, however, usually occur in persons 40 to 50 years of age (though, like senile dementias, they can occur in persons over 65). These diseases are characterized primarily by personality disintegration and intellectual deterioration.

Both Pick's disease and Alzheimer's disease are clinically similar except that Pick's disease is characterized by lack of initiative, Alzheimer's by aggression. Both diseases are inevitably fatal.[1]

Physical Dysfunction
Parkinson's Disease

Parkinson's disease, a degenerative disorder of the central nervous system, is the third most common chronic disease (cerebral vascular disease and arthritis rank first and second respectively) of late life. Parkinsonism may be classified in two ways: *symptomatic* (a result of cerebral arteriosclerosis, encephalitis, toxicity, or high dosages of the phenothiazines) and *idiopathic*.

Parkinson's disease is characterized by several physiological changes. In the extra pyramidal tract at the substantia nigra we find an increase of glial cells, a chemical deficiency, depigmentation, loss of neurons, and the appearance of Lewy bodies (intracyctoplasmic inclusions). In the basal ganglia of the brain stem there is cell loss and chemical deficiency. Researchers believe that Parkinsonism may be caused by the failure of the degenerating neurons in the substancia nigra to transmit dopamine (the precursor of norepine-phrine) to the striatum.[7]

Changes within the extra pyramidal tract are responsible for such characteristic Parkinson symptoms as rigidity, loss of balance, and tremor. Loss of dopamine transmission permits the cholinergic pathways to predominate. The following are specific characteristics commonly associated with Parkinsonism:

1. *Involuntary motion.* Parkinsonism tremor, initially involving the flexion and extension of the thumb and index finger, results in what is commonly referred to as "pillrolling." This type of tremor may also be found in the fingers, wrists, forearms, and ankles. It is most pronounced when the patient is at rest and increases with emotional stress or fatigue. On the other hand, it is absent during sleep and suppressed during activity.

2. *Rigidity.* This phenomenon, affecting both flexor and extensor muscles, takes two forms: *leadpipe* and *cogwheel.* Leadpipe rigidity refers to increased resistance throughout the entire range of motion when the upper and lower extremities are passively moved. Cogwheel rigidity occurs in a jerky intermittent manner; there is impairment of fine motor movements of the upper extremities (eg, buttoning becomes a more difficult task, writing becomes increasingly micrographic, and respiration becomes irregular and shallow). The typical Parkinsonism posture is displayed in flexion of the head, shoulders, hips, and knees, with the patient moving forward of the normal center of gravity. The patient also experiences difficulty starting to walk, but once walking is initiated, he moves increasingly in a more rapid manner and has difficulty stopping.

3. *Impaired motor function* (Bradykinesia). As the patient becomes less mobile, he moves in a more deliberate manner (often referred to as "freezing"). In the early stages of the disease, his gait is slow and there is reciprocal loss of arm movements. In the more advanced stage, his gait is shuffled and his steps smaller. Eventually his fine motor control is severely impaired.

4. *Dysfunction of the cranial nerves.* The ocular, facial, and oropharyngeal nerves cease to function appropriately. The malfunctions may take several forms: difficulty in swallowing, chewing, and expressing facial movements; disturbances of eye function such as convergence and oculogyric crises (ocular fixation in one position for a prolonged period); and dysfunctions of speech including decreased volume, monotonous tone, and poor enunciation.

5. *Impairment of equilibrium responses.* Patient loses his righting or protective reactions and is unable to maintain a standing balance.

6. *Disorder of the autonomic nervous system.* Dysfunctions within the autonomic nervous system include increased salivation, perspiration, bladder malfunction, greasy skin, intolerance to heat, and diminished peristalsis.

Medical treatment for Parkinson's disease involves a variety of drug therapies such as anticholinergics, antihistamines, Levodopa (displays undesirable side effects such as nausea and vomiting), and Sinemet (this combination of Carbodopa and Levodopa does not manifest unpleasant side effects).[8]

Joint Disease and Osteo-Disorders

Arthritis (from the Greek roots "arthron" meaning joint and "itis" meaning inflammation) is one of the most common and oldest of chronic diseases to plague elderly persons.** Although there are many kinds of arthritis, this discussion will focus on the types which most often involve the elderly—osteoarthritis, rheumatoid arthritis, and gout. A brief discussion of osteoporosis, which is not an arthritic disorder, will also be included.

Degenerative Joint Disease

Osteoarthritis, a noninflammatory degenerative joint disease, is extremely common among elderly people. It is a progressive disorder of the movable weight-bearing joints. During the course of this disease there is pathological deterioration of the articular cartilage and formation of new bone at the margins of the joint and in the subchondral areas.[9]

Primarily this degenerative process can be traced to such reasons as impaired blood supply, heredity, the "wear and tear" over the years which we associate with the aging process, a single severe injury (secondary osteoarthritis), continued minor trauma, and excessive strain and wear on specific joint areas (eg, desk workers may develop this disease in the neck and spine while obese people may develop osteoarthritis in the knees).[10]

Specific changes in cell cartilage, including 1) the loss of density which is exhibited by the presence of fibrillations (series of cracks)

**Webster's New Collegiate Dictionary. *Springfield. Mass. G & C Merriam Co, 1976. p 63.*

and 2) increased erosion (flacking of cartilage on its articular surface), usually cause the body to produce extra calcium in the form of osteophytes (boney spurs). This combination of osteophyte formation and cartilage degeneration often produces stiff and immobile joints. (A specific example is Herbeden's nodes, nodular enlargements of the distal interphalangeal joints found in many women with osteoarthritis.)

People with degenerative joint disease often complain that they experience stiffness and pain upon rising in the morning, during damp weather, after prolonged static positioning, and during periods of fatigue.

Medical treatment of this disease includes chemotherapy (aspirin is the drug of choice); local support when necessary (splints, canes, crutches); heat; specific exercises designed to correct muscle atrophy; and surgical procedures such as debridement, arthrodesis (joint fusion), arthroplasty (new prosthetic articulating surface), osteotomy (section of a bone is used to alter weight-bearing surface), and total joint replacement.[9]

Rheumatoid Arthritis

Rheumatoid arthritis, a disease process that can occur at any age, usually begins within the joints as an inflammation of the synovial area. It is characterized by edema, vascular congestion, cellular infiltrate, and fibrin exudate of the synovium. Usually the synovial fluid decreases in viscosity and becomes turbid. During the course of this disease there is a distinctive tendency towards spontaneous exacerbation and remission.

Although there is no specifically known cause for rheumatoid arthritis, many theories exist. Some scientists believe it to be caused by infectious agents (mycoplasma and viruses), others by immune mechanisms (such as antigen antibody complexes—the interaction of IgG and rheumatoid factors), and still others by Lysosonial enzymes.[9]

The pathological process of the disease involves the following changes: the blood vessels supplying the synovium become inflamed, the synovium thickens and proliferates, and more synovial fluid is secreted. As this synovial growth increases, the entire joint area becomes edematous and extends over the cartilage. The synovium and the surface of the articular cartilage then become a thick, sticky, and fibrous layer (pannus formation). As the process continues, cartilage may be destroyed, bone formation may occur (ankylosis), and there may be adhesions between the joint surfaces. This type of pathology can produce a totally immobile joint or instability and partial dislocation of the joint.[10]

At the onset, the symptoms of rheumatoid arthritis are insidious (aching and stiffness are usually poorly localized to the joints). As the disease progresses, many patients complain of stiff joints upon awakening. Joints of the hands (particularly the proximal interphalangeal and metacarpophalangeal joints), the feet (particularly the metatarsophalangeal joints), the wrists, elbows, knees, ankles, and subtalar joints are frequently involved. Tenosynovitis is extremely common, with the extensor and flexor tendon sheaths about the wrist being most often affected. Carpal tunnel syndrome (median neuropathy) may also be manifested. Joint involvement in rheumatoid arthritis tends to be bilaterally symmetrical.

The disease often results in serious deformities. Fixed deformities are caused by the inflammation and subsequent fibrosis in ligaments, capsule, and musculotendinous apparatus. Subluxation (slipping of one articular surface past another) is usually caused by erosion of bone and cartilage as well as the destruction of supporting soft tissues (such as ligaments and joint capsule). Characteristic hand deformities include ulnar drift, subluxation of the metacarpophalangeal joints, enlargement of the proximal interphalangeal joints, boutonniere deformity (flexed proximal interphalangeal joint is forced through the extensor hood), and swan neck deformity (contraction of the intrinsic hand muscles producing hyperextension at the proximal interphalangeal joint and flexion at the distal interphalangeal joint).[9]

Medical treatment of rheumatoid arthritis includes chemotherapy (aspirin being the most effective drug) and a variety of orthopedic and surgical procedures (splinting, insertion of a metal cup in the hip joint, complete replacement of joints by artificial devices, tendon repair, and synonectomy).

Gout

With gout, blood deposits of uric acid crystals form in the kidney, various joints, and certain cartilages. These chalky deposits (tophi) are directly caused by an increase in uric acid in the blood.

The disease is characterized by recurring attacks of acute painful swelling in a variety of joints, most commonly the big toe (50% of cases) and the elbow. It is more common in men (85%), the usual period of onset being after age 40.

The following factors are believed to be instrumental in precipitating gout attacks: injury to the joint, eating food that contains excessive amounts of purine (such as rich meats, duck, goose, sweet breads), excessive alcohol, and physical and mental stress.

Treatment involves the control and prevention of future attacks as well as the long-term reduction of hyperuricemia. Both can be accomplished through chemotherapy using uricosuric agent drugs (such as colchicine, phenylbutazone, and oxyphenbutazone). These drugs aid in the elimination of excessive uric acid. Appropriate diet is also recommended (food with little purine or alcoholic content).[10]

Osteoporosis

A common problem among elderly persons, osteoporosis is characterized by the thickening of the bone cortex, a compensatory reaction that occurs on the periosteum (outer layer of the bone). These new bone deposits are responsible for changing the actual shape of the bone (that is, the angle between the femur's neck and the shaft may change from an obtuse to a right angle). Because of these structural changes, the older person becomes less able to withstand trauma, and is therefore predisposed to an increasing amount of bone fracture.[11]

Heart Disease

Heart disease, the number one cause of death in the United States, actually covers a heterogeneous group of diseases which affect the heart. It can be broken down into three categories: cerebrovascular disease, diseases of the circulatory system, and cardiovascular-renal diseases.

Cerebrovascular disease is attributed to vascular lesions that affect the central nervous system. These lesions are generated by ischemia (infarction of the brain that may be caused by atherosclerosis, thrombosis, or cerebral embolism) and cerebral hemorrhage.

Diseases of the circulatory system include the following disorders: rheumatic fever, chorea, rheumatic valvular disease, rheumatic endocarditis, myocarditis, arteriosclerotic and degenerative disease, acute and subacute endocarditis, acute myocarditis, acute pericarditis, functional diseases of the heart, hypertensive heart disease and hypertension, arteriosclerosis (atherosclerosis of the coronary arteries which can manifest itself as myocardiac infarction, angina pectoris, coronary insufficiency, sudden death, congestive heart failure, and cardiac arrhythmias), aneurysms, peripheral vascular diseases, arteriol embolism and thrombosis, and diseases of the veins.

One of these diseases, arteriosclerosis, is a primary disorder that affects many older people. Arteriosclerosis is a generic term that refers to a number of different conditions which cause hardening of the arteries. Atherosclerosis (from the Greek "athera" meaning porridge and "sclerosis" meaning hardening) is one of these conditions: the center of a fibrous plaque in the wall of an artery is filled with a greasy "porridge-like" material. This chronic disease begins in childhood and progresses with age. Myocardial and cerebral infarctions, presently the most common immediate causes of adult death in the United States, are complications of atherosclerosis.

Cardiovascular-renal diseases involve a combination of heart disorders (that is, hypertensive heart disease) with other diseases such as chronic nephritis and renal sclerosis.

The exact cause of heart disease has not yet been determined, but the following items are considered risk factors: genetics (hereditary factors), gross obesity, social and psychological stress, high serum cholesterol levels, elevated arteriol blood pressure levels, smoking, and such disorders as diabetes mellitus, hypothyroidism, myxedema, and rheumatic fever.

Medical treatment of heart disease varies with the specific problem. Chemotherapy in the form of anticoagulant drugs can be effectively used to help prevent complications of acute heart attacks (thrombosis and embolism). Numerous drugs are also available to help lower blood pressure levels. Surgical treatment includes replacing damaged arteries with artificial ones, bypassing damaged segments, and in rare cases, transplanting the heart itself. Mechanical devices (such as alternating-current cardiac defibrillators, cardioverters, direct-current cardiac defibrillators, and cardiac pacemakers) are used to restore the heart rate to a more normal beat.

Cerebral Vascular Accident (Stroke)

Stroke can result from any of three major factors:

1) occlusion caused by thrombosis (clotting of the cerebral vessel).
2) rupture of a cerebral vessel caused by high blood pressure or a flaw in the vessel wall (which results in an aneurysm, a sac that presses on the brain and threatens that organ with hemorrhage).
3) occlusion caused by an embolism (a fragment of a clot that becomes dislodged from the heart or blood vessels and plugs the cerebral vessel).

Thrombosis and embolism account for the majority of cerebral vascular accidents.

All of these factors result in an inadequate supply of oxygenated blood to parts of the brain (the brain demanding more than one fifth of all blood pumped from the heart). The newly developed CAT scanner is helpful in determining specific areas of brain dysfunction.

Warning episodes of stroke include brief attacks of speech loss, weakness of the limbs, staggering, and loss of consciousness.

Medical treatment of the stroke patient involves the use of high oxygen pressure chambers, blood vessel surgery, and chemotherapy to improve blood circulation and control fat metabolism and hypertension. Cerebral vascular accidents can cause massive impairment of intellectual and motor functioning (aphasia and hemiplegia).[12]

Aphasia

Aphasia, a symptom-complex condition, is now believed to be the direct result of a lesion to the left side of the cerebral hemisphere. This usually results in decreased language competency. Aphasia can be classified as *receptive* and *expressive*.

The receptive aphasic has difficulty comprehending spoken (auditory aphasia) or written (alexic aphasia) symbols. Specifically, he confuses words that sound alike when spoken such as *moat* and *boat;* he indiscriminately mixes words that are associated in experience and meaning such as *sky* and *blue* (semantic confusion); he suffers a reduced naming vocabulary and reading vocabulary (his reading further hampered by associated errors and perceptual confusions); and he has difficulty understanding abstract words *(hope, peace)* as well as difficulty comprehending words which indicate relationships *(if* and *but).*[13]

In expressive aphasia the individual is not able to adequately express his ideas in writing or speech. His written and spoken vocabularies, especially nouns, are reduced and impoverished. When writing, he may reverse letters, confuse similar letters, and exhibit poor phonetic spelling. His speech often consists of telegraphic utterances, for example, "eat apple," "drink tea." Since he has difficulty utilizing words that express conditions, relationships, and qualities, his sentences are often agrammatic. He may also exhibit a specific impairment in his speech delivery—hesitancies, slowed or quickened speech rate, faulty word pronunciation, and reversal, omitting, and incorrect usage of sounds or syllables.[14]

Pure receptive and expressive aphasia rarely exist. Instead, aphasic disability is associated with multiple dysfunction of language modalities such as comprehension of spoken language, reading, writing, and speech. Specific perceptual-motor or sensori-motor deficits may be superimposed upon this condition.[13]

Cancer

"... Cancer is a term applied to a group of diseases having in common the transformation of normal body cells into abnormally growing parasitic cells."[12]

The basis of the illness is the cancer cell. While there are numerous known agents that can transform healthy cells into cancer cells, there is as yet no known single cause for the transformation. (Some scientists believe the answer to be a virus.) Scientific studies show that cancer cell nuclei differ from normal cell nuclei in several respects: they are larger, vary in shape, do not adhere to each other as much as normal cells, and they show deviations in the number and appearance of chromosomes.

Diseases of the cancer family have certain common characteristics: invasiveness into surrounding tissues, metastasis (transfer of a part of a cancer to another body part), hemorrhaging in tumor areas, a wasting away of the host, deviations in structure and function from the normal, and occurrences of superimposed infections.

The most common sites for cancer in males are the skin, lung, prostate, large intestine, stomach, rectum, and bladder. Common female cancer sites are the breast, cervix, uterus, large intestine, corpus uteri, ovary, stomach, and rectum.

Many factors can precipitate the disease: unnecessary exposure to ionizing and ultraviolet radiation, non-hygenic measures in occupations which involve exposure to cancer-producing dust and chemicals, late identification of probable precursors (cervical cancer, for example, can be detected and treated in its early stages using uterine cytological tests), excessive exposure to tobacco, and heredity (sex, age, family history).

Medical treatment of this condition involves the surgical removal of the cancerous areas, radiation therapy, and chemotherapy.[12]

Emphysema

Emphysema is derived from the Greek word "emphystma" which means body inflation.‡ With this disease the passages leading to the lung alveoli (air sacs), the smaller bronchioles, and the blood vessels become constricted. Little oxygen can reach the alveoli. Consequently, carbon dioxide accumulates in the air sacs. There is a constant decrease in arterial saturation of oxygen. As the disease progresses, the lung alveoli become enlarged and their elastic tissue is lost. There is a definite decrease in vital capacity and maximum breathing capacity. In the most severe cases there may be brain damage and an enlarged, weakened heart.

Many physicians believe that emphysema originates with a bronchial infection.[15]

‡Webster's New Collegiate Dictionary. *Springfield, Mass, G & C Merriam Co, 1976, p 373.*

Diabetes Mellitus

Diabetes mellitus can be defined as the body's inability to metabolize carbohydrates normally. These carbohydrates, in the form of glucose, accumulate and result in an increase of blood sugar. Eventually, this leads to sugar in the urine.

The exact cause of diabetes is unknown. Originally it was believed that diabetes was the direct result of deficient insulin action. However, recent research indicates that diabetes may be a multihormonal disturbance.[16] Specifically, researchers in San Francisco have been able to produce human insulin by means of genetically engineered bacteria, recumbinant DNA (deoxyribonucleic acid) technology. Large scale production is expected within the next five years.[17]

Though its cause is unknown, the disease can be closely related to four factors: obesity, heredity (according to Mendelian laws of inheritance), stress and urbanization, and arteriosclerosis (arteriosclerosis is responsible for 60% of all diabetic deaths.)

Some symptoms of diabetes include repeated infections, gangrene, early cataracts, pruritus (especially in the genital areas), undue exhaustion, impotence, extensive pyorrhea, and sudden refractory changes in the eyes.[18]

At present, treatment includes insulin therapy, cleanliness, and a measured balanced diet that is low in calories and high in nutrients. Although there has been much interest in the use of oral hypoglycemic agents such as Orinace, insulin remains the most effective form of chemotherapy. (Insulin is a purified hormonal extract of the Islands of Langerhans, developed by Bunting and Best in 1921.)[16] To avoid insulin shock, the diabetic must account for an increase in exercise or routine by a corresponding increase in his between-meal intake.[19]

If this disease is not treated, diabetic acidosis (coma) will result. This usually develops slowly (a period of hours). The symptoms, in their progressive order, include increased urination and thirst; drowsy restlessness; loss of appetite; abdominal symptoms of nausea, vomiting, pain; increase in temperature; Kussmaul respiration (hyperventilation with deep, regular sighing); dry skin; beef-red tongue; acetone on breath; rapid heart beat; and finally, unconsciousness. Bed rest, forced fluids, insulin, and cleansing of the bowels are the primary forms of treatment.[18]

Occupational Therapy And
Its Relationship To Disease

Since most older people experience at least two chronic diseases simultaneously, it is essential that therapists acquire a firm knowledge base of the diseases most prevalent among them. Understanding the progressive characteristics of these diseases is paramount in implementing and enforcing appropriate, substantive programs.

For example, an elderly housewife, diagnosed as having arteriosclerosis and diabetes, is recommended for instruction in work simplification techniques. An alert therapist, aware of her double difficulties, will introduce her to energy saving methods as well as instruct her in aseptic techniques.

Multidisorders also require that therapists be aware of the precautionary measures associated with the involved diseases. For example, a retired carpenter, suffering from emphysema, has been diagnosed as depressed. Because of his former skills, sanding a woodworking project would seem the therapy of choice for his depression. However, the accumulation of dust particles this project involves would severely aggravate his emphysema. Instead, the aware therapist interests him in another skill project, such as copper tooling, which has no contraindicated component.

Competent and efficient geriatric specialists are needed to administer appropriate treatment programs that encompass an understanding of the total patient. Continued study of disease and its corresponding treatment methods and modalities is necessary if this "whole person" approach is to become an effective reality.

6

Treatment Programs and Techniques

The biological, psychological, and socioeconomic losses that occur in aging as well as the variety of chronic diseases that plague the elderly are the foundation for therapists' awareness that this population segment is indeed in need of thoughtful, meaningful, and mature approaches.

Since occupational therapists are trained in the restoration of an individual's cognitive, emotional, and physical functioning, it is our obligation and mandate to provide treatment that is responsive to each consumer/client/patient problem.

Perhaps the most important aspect to remember about treatment is that the consumer should be involved as much as possible with his treatment program from its inception. Therefore, the therapist should recognize the patient's personal goals as well as clarifying the rationale for treatment. In this way, the client's motivation, an essential part of any treatment program, can be kept at a maximum. In treatment, the therapist has several roles:

1) to entice or interest the consumer to participate in his treatment program,
2) to provide appropriate and meaningful treatment that has achievable goals,
3) to alter treatment as necessary to the client's needs.

Included in this chapter is a diversified number of treatment techniques and programs that are available to the geriatric specialist. When appropriate, literature relating to the topic and other types of information will be suggested.

Reality Orientation

Many elderly clients in long term care institutions experience a multitude of cognitive, emotional, and physical impairments. The symptoms most often associated with these conditions include confusion, anxiety, depression, social withdrawal, disorientation, emotional liability, impaired judgment, impaired recent memory, inability to attend to self-care needs, difficulty communicating and socializing with others (tendency to isolate one's self from others), uncooperativeness, lack of self-confidence, and lethargy.

In 1958, Dr. James Folsom initiated the reality orientation technique at the Winter Veteran's Administration Hospital in Topeka, Kansas. It was later refined at the Veteran's Administration Hospital in Tuscalossa, Alabama in 1965.

Reality orientation is based on the assumption that repeated basic information (client's name, place, time of day, day of week, date, name of the next meal, and special events) can reinforce learning and ameliorate disorientation and confusion.

This type of program can be initiated by any staff member, family member, or volunteer who comes into frequent contact with the client. Formal reality orientation classes usually consist of four or five class members and an instructor. The classes should meet the same time every day at least five times per week. During this time, basic information can be reinforced by the following aids: reality boards (made of wood with movable slots so that appropriate information may be displayed), blackboards, plastic slates, bulletin boards, felt boards, mock-up clocks, name tags, calendars, and large bright pictures of food or other familiar objects.[1]

Classroom procedure includes the reinforcing of appropriate social skills as well as cognitive awareness (ie, appropriate salutation — "Hello, I am Mr. _____. What is your name?" — saying "good-bye" at the end of the session, and thanking the participant for attending). Initially, activities should be of a simple nature (identifying familiar objects, photographs, writing one's name on the blackboard), and they should gradually increase in complexity as the class members become less confused.

Within the classroom the following methods and procedures can be utilized.

1) A warm atmosphere (calm and friendly) is essential.

2) When addressing a class member, the instructor should always look directly at him and speak in a slow, clear voice.

3) It is important that each classroom member be given

adequate time and opportunity to respond.

4) If a class member does not know the answer to a question, the instructor should always tell him the answer and then ask the client to repeat it.

5) Immediate recognition and reinforcement of correct responses (such as "that's fine") are paramount ingredients of this program.

After the client has completed the basic reality orientation course, an advanced course, consisting of spelling, reading, math, writing, and discussion on current events, may be initiated.

Upon completion of the formal reality orientation program, graduation exercises are held. At this time a diploma (inscribed with the participant's name and graduation date) stating that the client has completed the prescribed reality orientation course is presented to him at a special graduation ceremony. The hospital nursing home administrator and staff, as well as friends and relatives, should be invited to attend.

Twenty-four hour reality orientation (informal reality orientation) takes place at the same time that the formal program occurs. This consists of improving the client's awareness of person, time, and place at any time a staff, family member, or volunteer have contact with him.[2] The following is an example of informal reality orientation:

Mr. X is found by the aide walking in the corridor at 1:00 A.M. The staff member states, "Mr. X, it is now 1:00 in the morning. Is it difficult for you to sleep? Here is your room and your bed. Your name is on your bed." The aide points to the name on the bed, reads it, and states, "It is time to rest now."

Attitude Therapy

Attitude Therapy, a consistent rehabilitative team approach, is helpful in reinforcing desirable behavior and eliminating undesirable behavior. This approach is often used in conjunction with reality orientation programs. It involves five major attitudes that are to be used with five types of behavior patterns. The professional team decides what attitude would be most effective with an individual client. Everyone coming into contact with this client

63

would then utilize the designated attitude. The therapeutic attitudes include active friendliness, kind firmness, passive friendliness, no demand, and matter-of-fact.

1) **Active Friendliness**—This attitude is most frequently prescribed for patients in reality orientation. It is most successful with older persons who are withdrawn and apathetic. Active friendliness is a supportive ego-building attitude that provides feelings of self-worth and accomplishment. The therapist should seek the client out (on a one-to-one basis) and sincerely praise him for his accomplishments.

2) **Kind Firmness** — Depressed elderly persons usually respond to this approach. The therapist should help the client focus on something else besides his own unhappiness. When using kind firmness, it is important that the client know exactly what is to be done and that the therapist expects his requests to be completed.

3) **Passive Friendliness** — This approach is useful for older persons who are suspicious and frightened by closeness and active friendliness. The therapist should wait for the client to make the first move and then respond by showing his interest and concern.

4) **No demand** — Older people who are distrustful, tearful, and experience global anger, respond best to this type of approach. Although activities and friendship are offered to these individuals, the resident should be made aware that the only thing that is expected of him is not to hurt himself or others.

5) **Matter-of-fact** — This attitude is prescribed for residents who demonstrate character disorders, anxiety reaction, psychosomatic manifestations, and seductive and manipulative behavior. The therapist should respond to the client's pleas, complaints, and maneuvers in a reality-based calm, consistent, and casual manner.[1]

Remotivation

This technique is usually begun following the successful completion of a reality orientation program. Its purpose is to encourage moderately confused older individuals to become more interested in their surroundings and environment by focusing their attention on simple, objective topics that are not related to the person's emotional problems. Another goal is to strengthen the client's ability to communicate and socialize with others. A remotivation series generally continues for 12 weeks (one session per week — each session from 30 to 60 minutes long). The group size consists of five to twelve residents. Each session makes use of a five point outline.

1) *Climate of Acceptance* — The remotivator greets each member by name and thanks him for attending. Pleasant appropriate remarks relating to the well-groomed appearance of some members (ie, "Mrs. Z, that is a very cheerful dress you are wearing"), and comments about the weather or news generate an atmosphere of warmth and acceptance (five minutes).

2) *Bridge to Reality* — A topic concerning the "real world" helps the participants to focus their interests upon the world in which they live. Three techniques may be utilized to introduce the topic: 1) poetry, quotations, or newspaper articles, 2) bounce questions, and 3) visual aids. The remotivator should encourage the group members to participate in the discussion or read portions of a poem or article (15 minutes).

3) *Sharing the World We Live in* — The remotivator stimulates discussion in a specific direction by utilizing a list of ten or twelve objective questions that have been prepared in advance. The therapist should be knowledgeable about the discussion topic and be able to answer any questions that are to be a part of the program (15 minutes).

4) *Work of the World* — The objective of this part is to encourage the resident to think about work in relation to his own being. Discussion concerning past tasks that the client has performed as well as current activities that he might be involved in are helpful (15 minutes).

5) *Climate of Acceptance* — The final section includes a time for the remotivator to review the high points of the discussion, announce the time and date of the next meeting, and express his appreciation to the group members for attending (five minutes).[1]

Opportunities for Increased Learning

For those older persons who display a minimal amount of confusion, there are other types of group interaction programs that can be utilized to stimulate greater cognitive and social awareness. News clubs, fashion clubs, sports clubs, literary review groups, travel interest clubs, and history clubs are topical groups that can foster discussions and social involvement. An eclectic group that discusses a variety of subjects is another approach.

An atmosphere where learning is expected generates a conducive climate for positive reflection and the development of the self. During the discussion period certain attitudes and skills are essential if communication is to take place:

1) The ability to listen (the ability to assess what is being said and to discriminate and analyze the important issues from the nonimportant issues).

2) The ability to understand and respect another person's viewpoint.

3) The ability to express one's own point of view so that others can comprehend the speaker's intent.

At the beginning of each meeting (as in any normal social situation) the participants introduce themselves. A light refreshment may be served to provide a relaxed, pleasant atmosphere. Experience has shown that the optimum size group appears to be from five to twelve members. Specific goals that can be achieved are:

1) the development of concepts in communication,
2) the development of friendships,
3) to provide a forum to stimulate thinking,
4) to emphasize constructive thinking by means of a classroom model.

Important to the older person's sense of self is the supposition that elderly people can be considered capable of learning and achieving in the present and with expectation of future achievement.

The following list of books and magazines can be useful with these groups.

Books

Carson R: The Sense of Wonder. New York, Harper & Row Pubs Inc, 1965.
Cooke A: America. New York, Alfred A Knopf Inc, 1974.
Merle S (ed): Vacation Land U.S.A. Washington DC, The National Geographic Society, 1970.
Sherman D (ed): The Best of Life. New York, Time-Life Books, 1973.

Steichen E: The Family of Man. New York, The Museum of Modern Art, 1955.

Magazines

Donovan H (ed): Sports Illustrated. Chicago, Time-Life Inc.

Grosvenor M (ed): National Geographic. Washington DC, The National Geographic Society.

Thompson E (ed): Smithsonian. Washington DC, Smithsonian Associates.

Programs that provide opportunities for increased learning act as agents that positively affect the emotional and cognitive well being of elders. Therapists should consider learning to be an essential and normal part of the life process. When given the opportunity to participate in meaningful group settings, elderly people can achieve a more intense awareness of themselves and their environment.

The Life Review

The life review, a natural and normal process, is utilized by many older persons as they become more aware of their approaching death. The therapist can enhance this process by incorporating specific techniques and methods, applicable towards self-reflection, into the client's treatment program. In order to do this, one must first understand the meaning of the process.

> The life review is conceived of as a naturally-occurring universal mental process characterized by the progressive return to consciousness of past experiences, and particularly, the resurgence of unresolved conflicts; simultaneously and normally, these revived experiences and conflicts are surveyed and reintegrated. It is assumed that this process is prompted by the realization of approaching dissolution and death....[3]

The characteristics of this process include a progressive and often spontaneous and unselective return to past experiences. It is a time to review unresolved conflicts and, hopefully, successfully reintegrate them. If there is no opportunity to resolve one's conflicts, an individual may become depressed, filled with guilt and anxiety, and become panic-stricken. On the other hand, successful reintegration of former conflicts can lead to the righting of old wrongs, a feeling of accomplishment and pride, a sense of serenity, and an acceptance of mortal life.

In older people the life review occurs in a number of ways, such as a tendency to reminisce, tell stories, and participate in mild nostalgia. Many elderly people will tell their life story to anyone who is willing to listen. Others will conduct a monologue without an audience. Whatever the case, it is extremely important that this process take place.

Health personnel should be encouraged to listen with care and concern to the reminiscences of the elderly. Reviewing one's past experiences is not a preoccupation with the self, nor is it boring, time-consuming, and meaningless. Instead, the life review represents a necessary and natural healing process, and therapists should do everything possible to encourage its usage.

Compiling family albums and scrap books as well as studying one's geneology are examples of methods which help to enhance the life review process.[4] Too often occupational therapists tend to discount the listening aspects of therapy as actually being helpful. Instead, their focus is often upon activities. It is paramount in this process that there be an interested and caring listener. Listening can be considered as much a part of therapy as making a splint, instructing activities of daily living skills, or creating a craft project.

Physical Conditioning Programs

The art of keeping physically fit has many benefits: the amount of hemoglobin to the red blood cells is increased, the skeletal tone is heightened, fat deposits are reduced, mineralization of the bones is stimulated, oxygen is used more efficiently by the muscles, the heart becomes better able to deliver a greater volume of blood per stroke and at the same time its capacity to maintain a longer recovery period between beats is increased, nerve regulation of the heart becomes more stable, liver and kidney function is enhanced, and the individual's ability to relax, control emotions, and tolerate fatigue are improved.[5] If a new drug were developed that could achieve all these things, local pharmacies would readily be depleted of their stocks in a very short time. It is no wonder that a lethargic, television-viewing America (of all ages) is currently enjoying a physical fitness renaissance.

Any individual participating in physical fitness conditioning activities should be cautioned not to over exercise. It is important for everyone to be aware of the "Safe Exercising Pulse Test." An individual should know his *resting pulse* (the average heart beat, taken three days in a row which is evaluated upon awakening, but before getting out of bed) and his *maximum pulse,* the fastest rate a heart can beat safely (this should be determined by a physician). The safe exercising pulse is established by subtracting the resting pulse rate from the maximum pulse rate. To insure that there is no overexertion, one should keep the heart rate within ten to thirteen beats of the safe exercising pulse. As a point of interest, Dr. F. Kosch found the maximum heart rate of seventeen men between the ages of 70 and 79 to be from 155 to 161.[5]

A recent study concerning Master Athlete Paul E. Spangler, a retired 77-year-old physician from California, demonstrates that an individual can consistently achieve well-being in late life. Dr. Spangler, a 1975 National AAU Master's class IV-b Champion (competition for athletes 40 years and older) in the 400, 800, 1500, 5000, and 15,000 meter races, underwent intensive physiological testing. Dr. Spangler's physical functioning exceeded those people of comparable age who are more sedentary; his physical condition was similar to other Master Athletes, and his functioning approached standards that are often achieved by much younger runners. Observable age-related decrements were noted in measures of maximal pulmonary ventilation, maximal oxygen consumption, and maximal heart rate.[6] This remarkable person demonstrates that while one can never be 20 at 77, an individual is capable of maintaining excellent health standards throughout his life.

When initiating an exercise program, the therapist should always receive clearance from the client's physician. As the program progresses, the participant's physical condition should be monitored by qualified health personnel. Some therapeutic goals that a generalized group exercise program can achieve are listed below.

PSYCHO-SOCIAL FUNCTIONING
1. Provide opportunities for tension release
2. Provide opportunities for the appropriate release of emotions such as anger, hostility, anxiety, fear, frustration, aggression
3. Foster social interaction skills, group cohesiveness, and a sense of security
4. Develop awareness of physical appearance (self-identity)

COGNITIVE FUNCTIONING
1. Improve attention span
2. Increase awareness of body parts
3. Improve the ability to follow directions and visual cues

PHYSICAL FUNCTIONING
1. Increase range of motion
2. Improve muscle tone
3. Improve flexibility, coordination, and balance
4. Improve gross motor and fine motor functioning
5. Improve functioning of the cardiovascular and respiratory systems
6. Increase kinesthetic awareness
7. Improve endurance

There are many factors to be taken into consideration about exercise programs: one should not confuse exercise and overexertion. Exercise programs should begin gradually and never reach a frenetic pace; to get the most benefit from each exercise, the participant should strive to achieve full range of motion and generally not exercise beyond the point of pain. There is a need for a consistent routine of time (many elderly people prefer midmorning), place, duration of each session (30 to 40 minutes), and number of sessions per week. While it is recommended that exercise be carried out daily, it has been noted that group exercising two or three times weekly and individualized exercising on the other days usually provides a reasonable compromise. There should also be a routine order of exercise (starting with loosening up postures—walking briskly, breathing deeply—and then including a variety of body parts such as scalp, facial and eyes, neck, shoulders, elbows, wrists, fingers and hands, abdomen and hips, upper back and chest, lower back, knees and hips, toes, feet and ankles) which will insure the most efficient and beneficial management of the program.[7] Specific progress can be shown by measuring joint range of motion, grasp, weight loss, and balance tolerance at the beginning and at the conclusion of each session. A graph charting this progress is also helpful.

It is vital that the program include exercise that utilizes all the joints of the body as well as the major and minor muscle groups. Persons using wheel chairs should not be excluded as many exercises can be done from a seated position.

To insure effective communication it is essential that the therapist speak clearly, give visual cues and or demonstrations when necessary, and explain the purpose of each exercise prior to the activity.

While equipment is not necessary, male participants (in particular) respond well to a gym-like atmosphere (basketball equipment, punching bags, exercise bicycles). However, it should be noted that isometrics or weightlifting (physical activity that develops the voluntary muscle groups by means of short, rapid, forceful movement) do little to enhance total body conditioning. In fact, there is evidence that this kind of stress on the muscle bundles during contraction has a tendency to impede circulation.[8]

Can a generalized exercise program be effective? Frekany and Leslie evaluated the flexibility of the ankle, hamstrings, and lower back of 15 female subjects (residents of nursing homes and participants of a Golden Agers Club whose ages ranged from 71 to 90) after a seven month's involvement in a weekly generalized exercise program (TOES, The Oaknoll Exercise Society). The results demonstrated a statistically significant (p. <.05 level) improvement.[9] The findings of another recent study (Stamford, Hambacker, and Fallica) indicated that significant cardiovascular and psychosocial improvements were noted in institutionalized geriatric patients who participated in an exercise program.[10]

The Senior Actualization and Growth Explorations (SAGE), an innovative experimental mental health program for elderly people in preventive mental health groups and in nursing and convalescent homes, utilizes a variety of exercises and training techniques such as Hatha Yoga, meditation, Tai Chi Chuan, relaxation, group breathing, foot massage, visualization discussion, guided imagery, gestalt dream interpretation, Feldenkrais exercises, biofeedback, and autogenic training. This program has been especially effective with depressed older people. Its stated aim is to restore vitality to the older adult.[11]

Exercises and related techniques that can be utilized by older adults are described and clarified in the following materials.

1) Administration on Aging. The Fitness challenge in the Later Years: An Exercise Program for Older Americans. Washington DC, US Government Printing Office.

2) Delza S: Body, Mind in Harmony: Tai Chi Chuan (Wu Style):

Ancient Chinese Way of Exercise. New York, Cornerstone Library Publications, 1972.

3) Devi I: Yoga for Americans. New York, The New American Library, 1968.

4) Frankel LJ, Richard BB: Be Alive as Long as You Live. Charleston, West Virginia, Preventi-care Publications, 1977.

5) Hornbaker A: Preventive Care. Easy Exercise Against Aging. New York, Drake Pub Inc, 1974.

6) Kalish A: SAGE (three video tapes). Clarmont Office Park, 41 Tunnel Road, Berkeley, California, 94705.

7) Leslie DK, Mchure JW: Exercises for the Elderly. Des Moines, Iowa, Univ Iowa, 1975.

8) Geriatric Exercise Manual. Norristown State Hospital Occupational Therapy Department. Norristown, Pa, 19401.

9) Royal Canadian Air Force Exercise Plans for Physical Fitness. Ottowa, Canada, 1962.

Physical conditioning may also be accomplished by participation in sports (swimming, ice skating, boating, tennis, golf, ping-pong), social events (square, folk, and ballroom dancing), and special organizations (bicycle clubs, nature hiking groups).

Physical Rehabilitation and Restorative Techniques

The purpose of this section is not to duplicate already existing rehabilitation and physical dysfunction books and manuals, but rather to explore existing treatment possibilities and recommend specific resources.

Exercise Programs for the Stroke Patient

Therapeutic exercise helps to maintain normal joint movement by putting joints through their full range of motion, by strengthening muscles, and by improving motions so that they can become more coordinated and automatic.

The therapist may initiate the program as soon as the attending physician has prescribed the range of motion therapy. During these passive exercises the therapist moves the patient (who is in a supine position, usually in his hospital bed) slowly and gently, but never forcefully, through the range of motion of the following joints: shoulder—flexion, abduction, and rotation; elbow—flexion, supination, and pronation; wrist—flexion/extension, ulnar/radial deviation; fingers—flexion/extension, abduction/adduction; thumb—flexion/extension and abduction/adduction.

Exercise programs that the client can utilize in the privacy of his own home include self-ranging exercises and exercises involving pulleys.

The purpose of a self-ranging exercise program is twofold: 1) to prevent the affected hand and arm from becoming stiff and painful, and 2) to improve dressing techniques of the upper extremity. It is recommended that these exercises be done at a minimum of one time per day and that each exercise should be repeated ten times. As a note of caution, the exercises should be performed only within the client's tolerance for pain. Self-ranging exercises are usually performed with the nonaffected hand supporting and moving the affected hand. These exercises, done in a sitting position, should include: shoulder—flexion, abduction, and external rotation; elbow—flexion and extension; forearm—pronation and supination; wrist—flexion/extension and ulnar/radial deviation; fingers—flexion and extension; thumb—abduction and opposition.[12]

A home exercise pulley program (this device could also be installed in a nursing home or residential center) involves obtaining some inexpensive but necessary equipment: two three-fourth inch single wheel awning pulleys, two five-eighth inch screw hooks, eight feet of nylon rope, and two seven-inch pulley handles. The hooks are secured 16 inches apart, and the client sits beneath the device in an armless, straight-back chair. Exercise consists of raising the affected arm by pulling down with the noninvolved hand and arm. The affected arm is slowly lowered. This should be repeated to increase tolerance, but never to the point of fatigue. If the pulley handles are softened and enlarged and a "hook" grasp (not "power" grip) is employed, this program can be adapted to serve the needs of arthritic patients as well.

Relaxing techniques done in a supine position with the eyes closed are also therapeutic, as a balanced program of rest and exercise is essential. Slow and deep breathing are helpful as well as focusing attention to each body part and "making" these parts "feel" (through concentrated thinking) that they are very heavy. Warm tub soaks, soft relaxing music, and a semidark room are all atmospheric approaches that promote relaxation.[13]

Informational Sources for
Treating Physical Restoration

An excellent resource that incorporates the entire spectrum of physical dysfunction is *Occupational Therapy Management of Physical Dysfunction*. This manual was compiled by Edwina Marshall for the Department of Occupational Therapy, School of Allied Health Professions of Loma Linda University, California in August of 1972. The exhaustive subject matter of this volume was not solely intended for the geriatric consumer. However, much of the material is pertinent to the care and treatment of the geriatric client. This extensive resource includes well-defined, clearly documented procedures, methods, diagrams, and evaluations of the following subjects: self-care, adaptive equipment and assistive devices, splints, positioning, evaluation of dysfunction (range of motion, muscle testing, general function test of upper extremities), exercise programs, orthopedic dysfunction (including programs of joint disease, guide for treatment of rheumatoid arthritis, hand deformities, construction of plaster hand resting splints, directions for a paraffin bath, dressing techniques, motion economy etc), peripheral nerve injury, sensory re-education, neurological conditions (low back pain, progressive disabilities), muscle re-education, progressive resistive exercises, activity analysis, neurological dysfunction and body image, and spinal cord injuries and burns.

The fifth edition of *Willard and Spackman's Occupational Therapy* provides an abundant amount of information regarding all aspects of occupational therapy programming, evaluation, and treatment. This 800 page volume should be an essential part of any practicing therapist's library.

Be O.K., Fred Samons Inc, (Box 32, Brookfield, Illinois 60513) is now offering numerous manuals and books that deal with hand splinting (dynamic and static), mobile arm supports, sensorimotor evaluations, chronic lung disease, physical dysfunction, home care services, consultancy, and hand rehabilitation, as well as manufactured equipment and devices.

Other companies that offer manufactured equipment and devices for the physically impaired individual are listed below.

1) Abbey Rents (also known as Abbey-Medical).
   Call toll free number for catalogue (800) 421-1170.

2) Cleo Living Aides
   3957 Mayfield Road
   Cleveland, Ohio 44121

3) Everest and Jennings
   1810 South Pontices Street
   Los Angeles, California 90025

4) Fairway King
   3 East Main Street
   Oklahoma City, Oklahoma 73104

5) JA Preston Corporation
   71 Fifth Avenue
   New York, New York 10003

6) Jaeco Orthopedic Specialties Co
   Box 75
   Hot Springs, Arkansas

7) GE Miller
   484 South Broadway
   Yonkers, New York 10705

8) Orthopaedic Supplies Co, Inc
   9126 East Firestone Blvd, Bldg R
   Downey, California 90241

10) Rolyan Medical Products
   14635 Commerce Drive
   PO Box 555
   Menomonee Falls, Wisconsin 53051

Parkinson Team Management Treatment Program

Specialized programs that involve a multidisciplinary approach are gaining momentum in a variety of institutions. In an article in the *American Journal of Occupational Therapy,* Judith Carlson Davis described a Parkinson team group program that includes an occupational therapist, a physical therapist, an occupational therapy aide, a physical therapy aide, a social worker, a consultant speech therapist, and a physiatrist.

There are four goals for this Parkinson Treatment Program:

1) counteract the effects of rigidity by maintaining or increas-

75

ing range of motion, preventing contractures, and improving posture;

2) increase motor function by improving gait and balance, preventing weakness from disuse, increasing reciprocal movements, promoting fine coordination, and improving self-care abilities;

3) improve speech and the musculature utilized in speech;

4) provide a stimulating environment that supports the patient and encourages socialization.

Evaluations were carried out at the program's outset and at three month intervals. Each program session is built upon three phases:

1) a warm-up period that consists of exercises to improve range of motion, reciprocality, and mobility—mat exercises, exercises using the parallel bars, and exercises that utilize a stationary bicycle;

2) a period involving activities for equilibrium and mobility that includes range of motion exercises for all major joints as well as emphasizing a particular body part for a given session, exercises utilizing facial musculature, and dynamic and static balance exercises;

3) the final phase of socialization and coordination activities utilizing group games such as hot potato, horseshoes, basketball, bean bag toss, frisbee, shuffleboard, wand passing, cotton ball blow, tic-tac-toe, and individualized programs involving perceptual tasks, dexterity boards, and tracing.[14]

Therapeutic Hand Management Programs

The human hand combined with the human brain have been the two major developmental characteristics that permit the human species to control and adapt the environment in order to form a productive and intelligent societal system.

Many older people experience a loss of hand mobility and productivity due to a variety of degenerative diseases and traumatic conditions. In order to create appropriate therapeutic techniques and devices that will improve the hand's usefulness, it is essential that the therapist know the functional position of the hand. (The wrist is in slight extension with the fingers moderately flexed. The thumb's metacarpophalangeal and interphalangeal joints are extended. There is opposition and abduction of the first metacarpal joint and the thumb is directly in line with the radius.)

Hand Splinting

Through the use of splints it is possible to improve hand functioning. Hand splinting prevents deformities (joint tightness and contractures); prevents increased muscle imbalance; protects weak musculature; encourages the return of function and facilitates the re-education of muscles; strengthens weak muscles; transfers power from one joint to another; acts as a substitute for permanently paralyzed musculature; gives support to a painful part on a temporary basis, thus, permitting motion of the unaffected, painless musculature; and helps correct deformities.[15]

E.M. MacDonald suggests the following types of splints to achieve specific therapeutic objectives:

1) the use of retaining splints to assist in the reduction of contractures and joint stiffness;

2) the use of functional splints to obtain the greatest amount of function from an upper extremity that exhibits minimum power and range of movement, to inhibit further deformities, and to prevent muscle wasting and shoulder stiffness;

3) serial splints (that are fitted to the palmer surface of the hand and forearm) to correct flexion deformities (these splints, made from plaster of paris orthoplast, may be adjusted continuously as the joint range of motion increases); and

4) resting splints to assist in holding the hand in a functional position as well as preventing pain and further deformity.[16]

The Hollis Approach to Hand Management

Irene Hollis recommends serial splinting (by means of foam rubber or plaster) and T-Foam splinting to prevent or decrease deformities and/or contractures in the older client. T-Foam splinting is helpful with the hemiplegic patient during the flacid phase. Because of the nonpressure prone characteristics of T-Foam, this method is beneficial in preventing decubiti and other types of pressure sores. The construction of the splint consists of T-Foam backed by cardboard (with adequate provision for thumb mobility) that is fastened with velcro attachments. The affected hand is gently placed between the two pieces of T-Foam.

Hollis consistently stresses the value of developing individualized splints for each condition as opposed to standardized commercially available splints. Further, she believes that therapists should be creative in their use of materials, and that many inexpensive items suitable for therapeutic adaption may be obtained at PTA and garage sales.

The management of edema is another problem that Hollis considers. Many older patients experience this condition. Edema can be controlled by 1) wrapping the affected hand with surgical gauze (squeezing at the tip and working down) and 2) tapping the involved area with a therapeutic pom-pom. This device is derived from banding metal that has a soft foam rubber attachment at the top. The patient's affected area is gently tapped with the device (distally to proximal).[17]

Experienced therapists of Hollis' stature are often available for speaking engagements. Occupational Therapy Associations or a group of individuals can act as sponsors for these learning experiences.

Exercises for the Arthritic Patient

Evelyn Rossky, OTR, has developed a unique material, Theradoh, that is beneficial for the arthritic patient as it offers a minimum amount of resistance and, therefore, the patient experiences little pain upon exercise. The formula for Theradoh is as follows:

1½ cups flour
½ cup salt
3 tbsp mineral oil
½ cup water (approximately)

Combine flour and salt and add oil gradually to make a soft dough. Dust the table lightly with baby talcum to prevent sticking when first used. (This adds a pleasant scent).*

Theradoh can be used with hand exercises involving gross and isolated opposition, gross and isolated finger flexion, finger abduction, gross finger extension, finger adduction, thumb extension and flexion, and wrist extension.[18]

*Formula used with permission of Evelyn Rossky, O.T.R., Moss Rehabilitation Hospital, Department of Occupational Therapy, Phila, Pa.

Joint Positioning, Protection and Energy Conservation

For patients who cannot tolerate a conventional splint, joint positioning is a viable therapeutic alternative. Irene Hollis presents many casual postures and positions that can help the patient improve his functioning. For instance, most patients with rheumatoid arthritis experience ulnar drift. When at rest, they lean on their hands with their fingers flexed beneath their chins. Thus poor positioning is reinforced, and greater ulnar deviation is encouraged. Instead, these people should be taught to extend the fingers and assume a position in which the chin is cupped in the palm while the wrist is extended. In this manner the fingers are encouraged to rest along the jawline, and the pressure then is towards the radial side. Walls and door frames can also be employed in obtaining wrist and finger extension.[19]

Joint protection is another very important concern for the arthritic patient. Some points on conserving joint mobility are listed below.

1) Avoid long periods of time in positions of flexion (bent knees, hips, elbows, and fingers). These positions can lead to deformities. It is imperative to never place a pillow under the knees. Instead, positions of extension should be encouraged.

2) Maintain good body mechanics. When rising from a chair (use a chair with arm rests), the patient's buttocks should slide forward with the knees together. The feet are then flat on the floor, and the patient should lean forward (the chin is lined up with the knees). The patient, positioning his palms on the arms of the chair, is then able to push off at the same time that he pushes up with his hips and knees).

3) Avoid using static grasp (writing, knitting) or sustained positions for long periods of time. Activities involving repetitive, tiring motions are also contraindicated (vacuuming, ironing).

4) Use the strongest joints (or body parts) available for any activity (eg, closing a drawer with one's buttocks instead of using wrist and fingers).

5) Avoid using a tight grip. Kitchen and workshop tools should have flat handles. Foam may be wrapped (as it enlarges and

softens) on the handles of tools that are used most often. Hold objects in a palm-to-palm manner. Moisture should be pressed out of sponges or handiwipes instead of twisting.

6) Avoid using ulnar deviating pressure on the fingers. When opening a screw top jar, one should lean on the lid of the jar with the palm and use shoulder motion. It is helpful to place the jar on a sponge cloth (or use a suction device) at the bottom of the sink to obtain appropriate stability.

7) Avoid using lateral pressure on individual fingers. For example, by fashioning a telephone dialing device and using it in an adapted manner (slip foam over a pencil and hold it like an ice pick), one is able to maintain therapeutic positioning.

Daily routine should consist of balanced rest and activity periods. The conservation of energy is paramount. Energy conservation can be defined as expending the least amount of energy to complete a task (eg, work simplification, page 90). Some examples include sliding objects instead of lifting, using wheeled carts, making use of nutritious convenience foods, and supporting the elbows on the table when combing one's hair.[20]

Another resource regarding programming for the arthritic patient is Jeanne L. Melvin's book, *Rheumatic Disease: Occupational Therapy and Rehabilitation.* Melvin describes rheumatic disease and its implications for occupational therapy, medical and surgical treatment, evaluation techniques, and occupational therapy modalities (including diagnostic criteria, the use of the polyethylene gauntlet splint, positioning, adaptive devices, etc).[21]

Development of Sensory Learning Skills

Low Vision

Although most older people have some form of vision difficulty, the majority do not lose their sight completely. For those who experience low vision problems there are a number of devices and adapted materials that are available: Optiscope enlargers (usually magnifies four times its size), plastic script guides, signature guides, hand magnifiers, elastic line writing guides, large print telephone dial guides, movable illuminated magnifier lamps, bath security rails, soap with rope through the center and adapted adult games (such as dominoes with prominent raised dots, checkers with round and square men that fit into sunken squares, and large print playing cards).

Other leisure materials such as large print books, talking books, newspapers, and magazines may be borrowed from the local library. Additional information may be obtained from the following sources.

1) American Foundation for the Blind
   Aides and Appliances Booklet
   15 West 16th Street
   New York, New York 10011

2) Be OK Self Help Aids
   Fred Sammons, Inc
   Box 32
   Brookfield, Illinois 60513

3) Hammocher Schlemmer
   147 East 57th Street
   New York, New York 10022

4) Subscription for the "Weekly Large Print New York Times":
   New York Times Bldg
   West 43rd Street
   New York, New York 10036

5) Subscription for large print "Readers Digest":
   Readers Digest Association, Inc.
   Pleasantville, New York 10570

There are a number of therapeutic environmental changes that can be utilized in institutions to assist older people who experience varying degrees of visual loss. Color coding (the door jams at an entrance of specific areas or the entire area itself could be painted in one color), deliberate use of visual boundaries, redundant cueing, large names on doors, large numbers on clocks, and large print calendars on the walls all help to orient the older individual to his environment.[22]

In the home, color coding, redundant cueing, and deliberate use of visual boundaries can also be used as well as large print labeling of frequently used items (spices, medicines). Whenever possible, the client should be instructed in organizing techniques for performance of activities of daily living. This might include an analysis of kitchen or cooking patterns that could result in a more meaningful and efficient arrangement of cooking and dining equipment.

Hearing Loss

It is normal practice to have an annual sight test, but uncommon for one to have an auditory examination on a regular basis (unless there is pronounced hearing loss). There are many problems associated with hearing loss. Auditory decline can lead to suspicious and paranoid behavior, depression, and social isolation.[22]

The Bell System offers specialized communications equipment that can be utilized by persons with impaired hearing: a bone conduction receiver; a code-com set, and numerous types of amplification mechanisms. The code-com set converts sound into sight signals by means of a flashing light and converts sound into touch symbols by means of vibration on a disc the size of a half dollar. Thus, deaf persons who are deaf only or deaf and blind can use this device.†

The following list contains suggestions for communicating with hearing impaired older adults.

1) Speak clearly and with moderate speed.

2) Do not shout.

3) The speaker's face should be clearly visible.

4) The speaker should have the client's attention before initiating any attempts at communication. The therapist should position himself so that he is directly facing the client.

5) Stand still while speaking.

6) Use visual stimuli whenever possible (gestures, written messages, pictures, and demonstrations).

7) Rephrase questions if the hearing impaired person does not appear to understand the original statement (some words seem very much alike when spoken, ie, *up* and *cup*).

8) Minimize loud background noises (papers shuffling, chairs scraping, radio or television continuously playing).

9) If the client wears a hearing aid, make certain that it is working effectively, ie, that the batteries and cord are operating appropriately, the aid is turned on, and that there are no disturbing sounds generated by the aid.[23]

If the client is an appropriate candidate, he can be instructed in the use of sign language.

†*Services for Special Needs. Bell Telephone, PE-161, July 1975, pp 4-7.*

Sensory Deficits

Leona Richman has developed a therapeutic sensory training and stimulation program that can be used in day centers, hospitals, and nursing homes. It consists of exercises and procedures involving the kinesthetic, tactile, olfactory, auditory, visual, and gustatory senses that orient the older individual to his environment.

Kinesthetic treatment approaches involve exercises that stress directionality, movement of body in space, and proprioceptive input. In the environment, adaptive devices such as grab rails and bannisters assist the elderly in dealing with kinesthetic loss. Treatment to encourage tactile recognition includes stimulation of the skin's surface (especially the hands with various objects and textures). The therapist explains the name of each object as the participant touches them. Objects may include sponges, various types of cloth, plastic, flour, metal and wood, etc. Tactile stimulation can also be a means of communication and expression of affect (massage, handshaking, hand holding, and hugging).

Auditory stimulation involves the use of a variety of sounds (ball bouncing, whistles, records, bells, clapping, etc). The therapist should initiate the program with two sounds and gradually increase these as the participants improve in their orientation status. During this type of treatment, clients are encouraged to make their own sounds (via clapping, humming, singing, and tapping).

Techniques used to stimulate the olfactory sense include identifying and exposing the client to a variety of odors (orange, mustard, mint, vanilla, etc). The most effective method is to present odors that are in direct contrast to each other, such as acrid smelling substances as opposed to pleasant or sweet-smelling items. Again, it is wise to initiate this program with two odors and gradually increase these as the participants become more oriented. As a note of caution, noxious or harmful items should never be introduced as many confused elderly persons may try to eat the items that are presented to them.

Gustatory stimulation involves the tasting of a variety of foods. It is helpful to begin with the presentation of well-liked familiar foods (eg, ice cream, pudding). Recognition of different taste sensations is easier when the foods that are presented have strong opposing flavors.[24]

While this type of sensory stimulation program was originally intended for group participation, a modified sensory training program may be successfully used on a one-to-one basis at bedside.

Programs for the Aphasic Patient

In Aphasia, a multimodality language disorder, the client may experience difficulty in comprehending spoken or written symbols or difficulty in expressing ideas (in either a written or spoken form). This language disturbance may be accompanied by distress, inappropriate affect (fear, anger, crying, euphoria, or screaming), frustration, and perseveration (inappropriate repetition of an activity or word after the original stimulus has gone).

The treatment of the aphasic requires a multidisciplinary approach which should include a physician, speech therapist, occupational therapist, physical therapist, nurse, and social worker. Appropriate language patterns in the aphasic can be enforced by the proper actions.

1) The therapist can provide the patient with appropriate words in a natural paraphrasing or modeling manner if he is experiencing difficulty expressing himself.

2) The therapist should provide continuing auditory exposure (without reaching a fatigue level) so that the brain can begin to compensate for damaged areas.

3) The patient should be encouraged to speak, and the therapist should praise all attempts at speech.[23]

If the patient's goal is to strengthen or renew visual perception and eye-hand coordination skills so that he may write or understand written symbols, it will be necessary to involve him in language preparatory programs. These include the ability to identify a position in space (this would involve the identification of a form's position regarding up, down, right side, and left side) as well as being able to identify a form against a background.

Although Dr. Maria Montessori developed a variety of educational methods and equipment involving the comprehension of number and language concepts primarily for use by preschool children, many of these tools such as sand paper letters and numbers, phonetic object picture cards, phonogram cards, cut-out letters, movable alphabet, number rods, and counters are useful in adult language preparation programs.

The Three Period Lesson (developed by Dr. Jean Seguin) that Montessori utilized is also helpful to the older adult with language disorders. It consists of three steps: 1) the instructor names the item as he points to it; 2) the client is asked to point to the correct object as the instructor names it; and 3) the client is asked to name the object as the instructor points to it.[25]

Other materials that can be utilized were developed for educational purposes. These include association picture cards, motor expressive language picture cards, logic cards, homophone cards, category cards, hononym cards, antonym cards, same or different cards, auditory perception training series, visual sequential memory exercises, visual discrimination flip books, symmetrical match-up cards, and spatial relationship cards. These are available from the following.

1) Developmental Learning Materials
   7440 NatChez Ave
   Niles, Illinois 60648

2) Special Resource Materials Catalog (Modern Education Corporation)
   Post Office Box 721
   Tulsa, Oklahoma 74101.

In *Perceptual Dysfunction in the Adult Stroke Patient: A Manual for Evaluation and Treatment,* Ellen Siev and Brenda Freishat have classified perceptual disorders into four categories: the apraxias, the agnosias, spatial relations syndrome, and body image/body scheme disorders. This book includes clear definitions, multiple evaluations, and pragmatic treatment suggestions.[26]

*Communication with the Aphasic Patient*** by Lynn Hill (RD #2, Barneveld, New York 13304) has additional information on treatment of the aphasic.

Treatment and Program Techniques
Management of Life Skills (ADL)

Being able to care for one's daily needs permits an individual to be an independent and viable human being. Since occupational therapy is strongly committed to providing treatment involving the improvement and restoration of an individual to his highest level of

**Hill L: Communication with the Aphasic Patient. Utica, New York, The New York State Occupational Therapy Association Papers, 1977.*

function (based upon his current assets), our participation in all types of activity of daily living programs is essential. Some of these programs should include grooming and dressing techniques, self-feeding programs, transfer techniques, cooking and menu planning, work simplification, development of avocational pursuits, and utilization of community resources (including transportation systems, social, intellectual, and nutritional community facilities and programs).

Grooming and Dressing Techniques

A person's appearance is related to how that individual views and values himself. If a person is no longer able to independently care for his own grooming and dressing needs, his identity and self-worth may come into question. The development of responsibility for self-care (increasing independent functioning), the improvement of self-identity and self-concept, as well as increasing appropriate awareness of one's body image (the self), contribute to feelings of self-worth.

Persons with physical disabilities need to learn special techniques so that they may become proficient in dressing themselves. For example, specific step-by-step instruction performed in a seated position that employs the principle of using the affected hand as a stabilizer (weight) and the noninvolved hand as a positioner and mover of the affected extremity is available to stroke patients. Detailed techniques (including illustrations) that demonstrate procedures for dressing—shirt, pants, short-leg brace, cardigan sweater (with dressing stick), may be found in *Occupational Therapy for the Stroke Patient.*[27]

Manufactured adaptive devices such as elastic shoe laces, long-handled shoe horns, long-handled bath brushes, suction denture brushes, velcro fasteners, long-handled hair brushes and combs, electric razor holders, metal rings on zippers, and suction bath brushes are available through suppliers (Chapter 6, page 75). These devices are helpful for people who have limited range of motion to groom and care for themselves. Since each patient is an individual with unique problems, the occupational therapist often needs to design and fabricate devices and equipment that are specific to his client's disability. To do this, the therapist must have a thorough understanding of his client's abilities and disabilities and the

86

intrinsic nature and capabilities of the materials that are being used (metals, velcro, plastics, etc).

Other grooming and self-care programs are instruction in shaving techniques, the appropriate purchasing and maintenance of clothing, application of make-up and instruction in hygiene techniques (including nail care, bathing procedures, hair care, and care and maintenance of the skin).

Self-feeding Programs

When a person loses the ability to feed himself, much of his autonomy and self-dignity is taken away. The occupational therapist can help him regain mastery of self-feeding skills by providing him with appropriate instruction in the utilization of specific feeding devices and equipment.

Manufactured items such as wrist supports with palmar clips, ball bearing feeders, offset suspension feeders, plastic food guards, swivel utensils, side cutter forks, suction holders, built up handle utensils, extension utensils, vertical and horizontal palmar self-handle utensils, utensil holders, offset spoons, wheel chair glass holders, flo-vacuum cups for drinkers in a supine position, and convalescent feeding cups are available from various supply houses (Chapter 6, page 75). Whenever possible, the therapist should try to design, fabricate, or alter individual feeding equipment; not only is an individualized feeding aid economical, it also is usually more effective and efficient. Sometimes adapting a simple item is all that is necessary. For example, a foam hair curler placed on the handle of a standard utensil is, in most instances, functionally equivalent to a ready-made built up utensil and at a fraction of the cost.

Transfer Techniques

As in feeding, self-mobility is linked with autonomy and independence. For a wheelchair patient the ability to transfer from bed to wheelchair and back, getting in and out of the bath, and mobility between wheelchair and toilet may mean the difference between being confined to bed or having some degree of control of self-movement and activity.

Being immobilized has many detrimental consequences such as increased tendencies towards the following conditions: thrombosis, hypostatic pneumonia, contractures, bowel and bladder problems, decubiti, stone formation, weakness, and emotional and mental changes (deterioration). Therefore, the therapist should make every effort to provide transfer and mobility training.[28]

In *Caring for the Elderly Patient at Home: A Family Guide (Activities of Daily Living)* complete instructions (with illustrations) describe the following transfer techniques:

1) bed to wheelchair—wheelchair to bed;
2) wheelchair to toilet—toilet to wheelchair;
3) bed activities (turning and sitting).

In general the hemiplegic patient utilizes his nonaffected extremity for strength, balance, and positioning and moving his affected extremity. (Cautionary note—wheelchairs must always be in a locked position before attempting transfer.)[29]

Cooking and Menu Planning

Planning menus and the art of cooking are combined skills that serve to enhance one's mastery of independent living. Too often older people who live alone will place little emphasis upon nutritional values. Instead, tea and toast often serve as a "quickie" meal. Because of these attitudes, older persons need instruction in nutritional planning. This should include an explanation of the different types of food that are needed daily to maintain a balanced diet. An understanding of the six major categories of food substances is necessary.

1) *Carbohydrates*—foods that provide the body with a quick energy source. For example, potatoes, starch, sugars, rice and spaghetti.

2) *Proteins*—major type of food that is involved in the replacement of body tissue; these are also an energy source. Proteins are found in such foods as fish, eggs, soy beans, and meat.

3) *Fats*—foods primarily intended to act as energy reserves. Oils, butter, and margarine are examples of fatty foods.

4) *Vitamins*—essential substances that promote proper body functioning. Unlike the other three categories, they are not involved in energy utilization.

5) *Minerals*—food factors that are needed to maintain appropriate body functioning. Examples of minerals include

calcium (found in milk products), iron, magnesium, potassium, and copper.

6) *Bulk Foods*—foods that maintain regularity and appropriate bowel functioning. Vegetables and cereals are examples of foods that supply the body with its necessary roughage.

Daniel S. Liang suggests the following items as a general diet plan for older persons.

Meat Group—two servings per day with a choice of liver, pork, beef, lamb, fish, poultry, and eggs (approximately four per week due to the high cholesterol count). Dried beans, dried peas, peanut butter, and nuts may be substituted.

Milk Group—two cups per day. Milk products such as cheese and ice cream are also included.

Fruit and Vegetable Group—four servings per day. Citrus and green leaf vegetables should be served at least four times a week.

Fats—butter and margarine twice daily.

Cereals and Bread—four servings per day. Whole grain breads and cereals are particularly helpful. Dr. Liang also recommends that generous amounts of water be served at every meal.[30]

Once the client's understanding and implementation of the value of nutritional menu planning is achieved, the art of cooking can begin. Therapeutic cooking should be a graded activity, starting with the making of a cup of coffee on a one-to-one basis and culminating in a cooking group experience that involves the cooking and serving of an entire meal.

Besides the actual knowledge and mastery of cooking skills that one can attain in this type of group activity, there are a number of other therapeutic goals that are equally important. These include improving the client's ability to perform tasks in the presence of others, to perceive and respond to group members' needs, to cooperate and share tasks with other people, to understand cause and effect relationships, to perform appropriate reality testing skills, to practice certain acceptable social graces and etiquette (manners), to follow directions and participate in decision-making procedures, and to function more independently so that community placement may become a reality.

Work Simplification

Work simplification techniques may mean the difference between dependency or organized independent functioning. Each activity or job needs to be analyzed to determine if any part can be eliminated. Almost every activity has three parts:

1) getting items in readiness for the activity;
2) the activity itself (motions should be analyzed to ascertain the most effective and efficient way to accomplish the job);
3) cleaning up and putting away of equipment.

Job analysis should include trying to find the answers to the following questions: *Is the job necessary? What is its purpose? Where is the best location for the activity? At what time should it be done? Who should do it?* and, *In what manner should it be done?* Guidelines for work simplification include:

1) eliminate all unnecessary details;
2) combine steps whenever possible;
3) when indicated, change body position and motions, tools, work place, equipment, sequence, raw materials, and finished products;
4) plan and organize work and adhere to the plan;
5) balance heavy and light tasks throughout the day and week;
6) have all work and storage areas within normal reach;
7) avoid fatiguing postures (bending, stretching, excess walking, holding);
8) slide objects instead of lifting and carrying;
9) whenever possible, let gravity work;
10) sit to work.[27]

Development of Avocational Pursuits

For those elderly people in the community who need a structured environment, the development of hobbies and other personal interests are paramount. Craft groups, photography clubs, gourmet cooking clubs, stamp collecting groups, and chess and bridge tournaments are activity groups that can be utilized to develop the client's personal interests. It is often the pursuit of avocational interests that prove to be the difference between a depressive "backward" rooming house experience and a day structured with meaningful activities. Occupational therapists have designed programs that combine avocational interests with community resources. One such program will be discussed in the next section.

Utilization of Community Resources

Elders who intend to return to the community should be instructed in how to find and use all available community resources. Many communities (often under the auspices of the local health and welfare council) maintain a booklet listing all the local services that are offered to older adults. These may include Dial-A-Ride (an individualized transportation system especially designed for elderly and handicapped persons), Senior Activities Centers (including group feeding, nutrition, craft and social programs), house-bound library loan programs (via the United States Mails), meals-on-wheels, R.S.V.P. (Retired Senior Volunteer Program), the local Area Agency on Aging (referral agency mandated to evaluate a client's problem(s) and ultimately see that he contacts the appropriate program, clinic, agency, or facility), efficient and energy saving banking procedures (the federal government will send social security checks directly to a client's bank), and friendly visitor and telephone companion programs.

The Neighborhood Extension of Activity Therapy (NEAT) Program, developed by Ellen L. Kolodner, provides opportunities for psychiatric patients to participate in a structured transitional-discharge activity program.[31] One of the program's major purposes is to foster feelings of efficacy and competency among psychiatric patients who are involved in the discharge process. Neighborhood Extension Activity Therapy assumes that many patients experience a great deal of difficulty utilizing their leisure time in a constructive manner. These periods of unstructured time often lead to the extinction of essential skills that the patient needs in order to interact effectively with his environment. NEAT uses a series of collaborative interviews between the therapist and client to ascertain the patient's specific activity preference. In this respect, the Interest Checklist of J.S. Matsutsuyu is instrumental in providing a comprehensive interest inventory.[32] Once the patient attends community activity programs, it is essential that supportive follow-up be provided. The consumer and the therapist contact each other on a weekly basis (by telephone or in person). During this time the therapist investigates and analyzes the client's life-style adjustment patterns. New activities or an activity configuration may be recommended. As the patient becomes more skilled in his use of activities, his feeling of competency and desire for independence deepens. Thus, there is less need for support, and gradually the former patient is weaned away from hospital interaction.

Client Determined Approaches to Treatment

The consumer revolution is just beginning. Greater numbers of citizens are questioning the quality of health care delivery systems within our nation. These Americans no longer fill the acquiescent, quiet patient role. Indeed, they want to know what their problems are and the how and why of treatment. Once the sole domain of the health professional, treatment has now become a cooperative venture between the patient and the therapist.

Even though a client may be limited in his ability to comprehend, every opportunity should be afforded to involve him in as much decision making activity as is possible. For those patients who are institutionalized in large state hospitals, this kind of concept can enhance, enrich, and give new meaning to their lives. Since many of these elders have few friends or family members who may be concerned about them, the employees (within the institution itself) need to assume a patient advocate stance. The Geriatric Occupational Therapy Program at Norristown State Hospital maintains that elderly chronic patients are capable, with support, of making decisions that affect their life situations. It is a self-determined atmosphere that aids in defeating institutionalized dependency and patronization.

Group direction, names, and purposes of each activity or club are discussed and decided upon by the program members and the therapist. Some of the therapeutic groups that have developed as a result of patients' specific interests are listed below.

Variety Club. In this group, individuals are encouraged to make projects for friends, family, or themselves. Arts and crafts modalities are used.

Friendship Club. These club members are concerned with the emotional and physical well-being of residents within their building. They protect the beautification of the environment (posters, hanging baskets), write to recently discharged members, and send get well wishes to patients who are in the local community hospital.

Garden and Ecological Club. The members of this group are involved in raising vegetables, indoor plant care, and flower arranging.

Cooking Club. This group's primary goal is to involve each member in the preparation, cooking, serving, and cleaning up of the dinner meal.

Grooming Club. The purpose of this club is to enhance one's personal appearance. These activities provide patients with opportunities for developing a sense of responsibility and caring relationships with each other, comprehension of cause and effect relationships, opportunities to improve eye-hand coordination skills and attention span, and opportunities for proprioceptive input and improved muscle tone.

There are three major program objectives that are associated with each club program: 1) the development of the self, 2) encouraging a sense of awareness of one's environment, and 3) developing effective, appropriate communication and social skills.[33]

Processes to Achieve Improved Sensorimotor Integration

Many of the residual long-term population of older patients within state hospitals are chronic schizophrenics. While Director of Rehabilitative Therapies at Arizona State Hospital in Phoenix, Lorna Jean King observed a number of postural and movement patterns that are typical of process schizophrenics.

1) The postural presence of a definite head to toe S curve.

2) The lack of a normal heel to toe pattern producing a shuffling style of gait.

3) A pronounced inability to raise the arms above the head.

4) An immobile head and shoulder girdle which is markedly manifested by the inability of most patients to tip their heads back.

5) The arms and legs are usually held in an adducted, flexed, internally rotated position.

6) The hand does not function in a normal manner—the thumb is adducted, the thenar eminence displays atrophy, there is ulnar deviation at the wrist, and a pronounced weakness of grip is noted.

7) Psychomotor retardation is present.

8) There is tension in phasic muscle groups and hypotonicity in the totonic (opposing) group.

It is hypothesized that defective proprioceptive feedback mechanisms (particularly the vestibular components) may result in an abnormal or poorly organized sensorimotor integration process.[34]

J.A. Ayres postulates that vestibular and tactile input performs a critical role in organizing and integrating sensory stimuli (primarily at the brain stem level).[35] Sensory input and integration is essential in developing appropriate visual size and form constancy and reliable localization of auditory stimuli.

King proposes that the lack of perceptual and auditory constancy, due to faulty sensory integration, may be a prime factor in producing hallucinations. She also hypothesizes that the schizophrenic's lack of sensorimotor integration is due to corticalized movement.

Treatment at Arizona State Hospital is focused upon the development of sensory integration. Many of Ayre's sensorimotor-integration treatment theories were adapted and incorporated into the Arizona Program.

It should be stressed that when working with an older adult, the patient's physical capabilities must be considered. Continual monitoring of the vital signs by health professionals and an awareness of the individual's safe exercising pulse rate are essential in determining the patient's endurance level.

King recommends these specific sensory integrative treatment approaches:

1) the motor process is focused upon an outcome rather than cortical planning;
2) the activities must be pleasurable;
3) incorporate as many ways of stimulating the vestibular mechanism as is possible (move the head in a plane through a significant distance);
4) activities that involve the bilateral use of tonic muscles should be included;

5) activities that integrate primitive reflex patterns are also recommended;
6) include pressure touch activities;
7) involve activities that have proprioceptive feedback from tendons and joints;
8) incorporate activities that utilize other aspects of sensory input (eye pursuits, awareness of form and space, color, texture and rhythm).

Balloons, beach balls, textured fabrics (terry cloths, velvet, burlap), nerf (sponge) balls, rhythm instruments, and parachutes are some of the equipment and materials used to perform these activities. Treatment goals for sensorimotor-integrative approaches include improved perceptual constancy, improved body image, effective and appropriate motor planning, and efficient nonfatigue producing postural patterns.[34]

Craft Modalities for the Older Client

The objective of this section is not to provide an exhaustive list of "how-to-do-it projects" but rather to introduce some inexpensive crafts that can be utilized by older men and women for therapeutic purposes. Included also are resources such as books, manuals, and magazines that are currently available to the geriatric practitioner.

Each project should have a therapeutic basis. Our mission as geriatric occupational therapy specialists is not to serve as arts and crafts instructors. Indeed, it is essential that the therapist's involvement be focused upon improving the individual patient's functioning abilities.

Since therapeutic craft approaches are often misunderstood by the patient and other health professionals, it is the paramount obligation of the therapist to seize every opportunity to explain arts and crafts treatment rationale (why a specific craft is being used and how it will improve a client's area of dysfunction) to all concerned persons.

Before an individual can begin to use a craft therapeutically, he must be aware of all the components that are involved within the specific activity. This would include analyzing four areas:

1) the intrinsic nature of the materials that are being used

(pliability, resistance, ability to be controlled, sensory qualities such as proprioceptive, gustatory, visual, auditory, olfactory and tactile);

2) the activity process itself (number of steps involved, the complexity of the activity, the type of directions that are needed, the preparation that is required);

3) the setting in which the activity will take place (location—at home or in the clinic, interaction—solitary, with another person or within a group);

4) the purposes or goals of the activity—craft activities are used for physical and psychiatric remediation.

The following discussion concerns specific examples of craft usage in Rheumatoid Arthritis. Its purpose is to demonstrate how craft therapy works. Activities are often selected to establish an initial rapport with the patient, to relieve anxiety, to discourage generalized immobility, and to prevent dependent behavior. If the hand is affected, mild activities that involve light pinch, lifting, and grasp (such as placing mosaic tiles in a tray) are indicated. Prolonged static positioning (as used in knitting) is definitely contraindicated. After the initial period of inflammation and pain has subsided, craft activities (ie, weaving—grasping the built-up handle of a loom while the patient is supported in splints) may be used to strengthen weak hand muscles.[36]

Therapeutic craft modalities can be used in a number of ways and have a wide range of restorative value. Treatment objectives that can be met through the use of crafts are stated below.

Psychiatric. Provide opportunities for self-identity, self-concept, and self-esteem; coping with success or failure; coping with fantasy and symbolism; comprehension of cause and effect relationships; appropriate outlets for anxiety, frustration, anger, tension, aggression, and hostility; opportunities to express creativity, originality, and need gratification; perception of the sexuality of self and others; opportunities for reality testing; and for tolerance in task or group situations.

Intellectual functioning. Improve ability to follow directions, make decisions, increase attention span, and awareness of body parts.

Physical restoration. Improve muscle tone, strengthen specific groups of muscles, increase range of motion, increase endurance, improve functioning abilities, and improve eye-hand coordination.

Other. Provides avocational or prevocational experiences as well as serving as an evaluative tool to assess physical and psychiatric functioning.

Although many projects need to be simplified (due to physical, emotional, or cognitive losses), they should never be childish. Indeed, craft activities can provide the older person with a sense of dignity and self-worth. For those elders who no longer work and who still want to be useful and productive human beings, crafts can offer a way to achieve this. The following project suggestions are inexpensive and suitable for older persons.

1. *Wood Collage.* Wooden scraps, obtainable at local lumber yards, can be glued on a masonite panel, sanded and stained to form wooden collage constructions.

2. *Clear Liquid Plastic Forms.* Clear liquid plastic (casting resin) is available in local hobby shops and wholesale houses in quantity or individual kits. A clear liquid plastic and hardener are poured into plastic molds. Shells, flowers, leaves, and stones may be incorporated into the design. A few words of caution—this type of project needs much ventilation and should not be carried out near a flame.

3. *Wooden Keepsake Boxes.* Wooden boxes with indentations on the lid are available at local hobby shops and wholesale houses. These boxes may be sanded, painted or stained. Tiles, decoupage, sequins, beads, shells, and stones may be used as decoration. Felt material may be pasted into the interior to form a lining.

4. *Scrapbooks.* Scrapbooks (made from construction paper) may be used to emphasize a particular theme such as sports, local and international news, holiday seasons, and food.

5. *String Art.* A board (scraps or purchases from a local lumber yard) sanded and stained serves as a background for nail designs. Brightly colored string (rubber bands can be substituted) are then placed around the nails to form a design.

6. *Wooden Cars, Trucks, Trains, and Trolleys.* Wood blocks (cutoff's of 2 x 4s may be obtained from local lumber yards) can be sanded, painted, and assembled into toy cars.

Popsicle sticks, spools, buttons, cardboard, and masking tape may be used to decorate the cars to make them more realistic. These make excellent gifts for schools and grandchildren.

7. *Mosaic Tile Plaques.* Tiles laid into a design are first glued to a masonite panel. Grout is then poured into the open areas. As it dries, a damp cloth can be used to wipe off excess grout. An orange or popsicle stick is useful in getting off any stubborn grout residue. These projects are suitable as wall plaques, trivets, and plant table-protectors.

8. *Paperweights.* Medium-sized rocks may be glued together (or used separately) to form a design or object (eg, ladybug, grasshopper, etc). The rocks are painted in appropriate colors that enhance the design.

9. *Safety Pin, Paper Clip, and Button Collage.* Household items such as buttons, safety pins, and paper clips are glued to a piece of wood, masonite, or heavy cardboard to form an interesting design. They may be sprayed with paint and then placed upon a contrasting background color.

10. *Placemats.* This project involves the use of washable wallpaper. Sample wallpaper books can usually be obtained free of charge in a local paint and wallpaper store. The samples are cut in the shape of place mats.

These projects represent a sampling of the types of simple, yet mature projects that are available. They may be used for personal needs or as gifts for the family and friends. Pride in one's accomplishments as well as being able to display one's skills to others can only lead to an increase in self-esteem.

Information regarding craft instruction may be obtained at libraries, hobby shops, department stores, and craft guilds. The "Y's", Adult Evening Schools, and some hobby shops will often offer classroom instruction in a variety of crafts.

There is an abundant supply of craft and activity books now available to interested persons. Some useful ones are listed below.

Andes E: Practical Macrame. New York, Van Nostrand Reinhold Co, 1971.

Black ME: New Key to Weaving. New York, Macmillan Pub Co Inc, 1975.

Clapper E, Clapper J: Pack-O-Fun Craft Projects: Make it Yourself with Odds and Ends. New York, Hawthorn Books Inc, 1972.

Coats and Clark's Sewing Book: Newest Methods from A to Z. New York, Western Pub Co Inc, 1967.

Enthoven J: The Stitches of Creative Embroidery. New York, Van Nostrand Reinhold Co, 1964.

Fish HU: Activities Program for Senior Citizens. West Nyack, NY, Parker Pub House Inc, 1971.

Gould E, Gould MA: Crafts for the Elderly. Springfield, Illinois, Charles C Thomas Pubs, 1971.

Kenny JB: The Complete Book of Pottery Making. Radnor, Pa, Chelton Book Co, 1976.

Macrame, Tricks and Treats. Phoenix, Arizona, Pappes Inc, 1975.

McCall's Books (needlepoint, soft toys, fashions, afghans, quilting, crafts, crocheting, knitting). 615 McCall Rd, Manhattan, Kansas 66502.

Merrill T: Activities for the Aged and Infirm. Springfield, Illinois. Charles C Thomas Pubs, 1967.

Pforr EC: Award Winning Quilts. Birmingham, Ala, Oxmoor Harris Inc, 1974.

Torbet L: How to Do Everything with Markers. New York, Bobbs-Merrill Co, 1976.

The following is a mailing list of craft supply companies:

Ceramics and Metal Enameling

1) Amaco
   4717 West Sixteenth St
   Indianapolis, Indiana, 46222

2) Bergen Arts and Crafts
   PO Box 381
   Marblehead, Mass, 01945

3) Stewart Clay Co
   PO Box 18
   400 Jersey Avenue
   New Brunswick, NJ

General Crafts

1) Griffin Craft Supplies
   P.O. Box 506
   Oakland, California, 94604

2) Horton Handicraft Co Inc
   PO Box 330
   Farmington, Conn, 06032

3) Magnus Craft Materials Inc
   304-8 Cliff Lane
   Cliffside Park, NJ 07010

4) S and S Arts and Crafts
   Colchester, Conn, 06415

Needle Crafts

1) Lee Wards
   Elgin, Illinois, 60120

2) Herschners
   Stevens Point, Wisc, 54481

Wool and Synthetic Yarns

1) Eliscu and Co Inc (Red Hearts Yarns, Coats and Clarks)
   10 Andrews Drive
   West Paterson, NJ, 67424

2) The Lily Mills Co
   Shelby, North Carolina

The United States is on the threshold of a new awareness that elders have just as much right to treatment as younger people. Life is precious no matter what a person's age. There are a host of relevant therapeutic techniques and programs that are available to the geriatric practitioner. As increasing numbers of Americans grow older, occupational therapists will have an opportunity to use their skills in promoting responsible health care for this population.

7

Coping with Death and Dying

Birth and death are two aspects of mortal existence that touch all humanity—the old, the young, the rich, and the poor.

It was written long ago, "What man shall live and not see death?" (Psalms 89:49)

Life and Death—A Comparative View

Modern western society tends to dichotomize death and life. Death is regarded as the cessation of biological and physiological functioning or, within a religious context, as the end of wordly affairs and the beginning of a new spiritual existence. Whatever the focus, the western world views the transition from life to death as abrupt, irreversible, and final.

In ancient times there was a limited life expectancy. Only a few people survived beyond the years of early maturity. The sight, sound, and smell of death were not insulated from communal life. There was no sense of possessing any control over the forces of nature. The extended family (tribe or clan) provided all the necessary strength and continuity. Individualism, as we know it, was not yet developed. The well-being of any one person was seen in relationship to that individual's performance and obligations to the group.

The modern conception of death is a world apart from ancient beliefs. Transposition, insulation, technology, and decontextualization are primarily responsible for these new attitudes toward death. Today's life expectancy is almost twice that of our ancestors. Because of this factor, our society tends to transpose death from an immediate and perpetual menace to one of remote possibility. Our way of life keeps us well insulated from the perceptions of death. Instead of the tribe or clan we have developed a technological team of death specialists (consisting of medical personnel, the clergy, death or grief counselors, and those trained in mortuary business and science—the "burying people"). Technological growth and scientific discovery have increased our power for reshaping and modifying our planet. Science is seen as the master and man the controller. No longer do we participate in a society built upon accepted dogma, lineage, or tradition. In previous times the individual relied upon deeply entrenched communal attitudes in his thoughts and practices about life and death. Today an individual is held responsible for his own ideas and actions.[1]

The American view of death and life, based upon a Judeo-Christian foundation, is different from that of other societies. The early Greeks believed that the living could visit the land of the dead. The Buddhists conceptualize life as continuous; death is seen as a time when the soul migrates from one form of life to another. In the Shinto religion, death is thought of as joining one's ancestors, who continue to consult with the living.[2]

Societal Attitudes

Death in our culture is distant, depersonalized, and camouflaged (eg, a cemetary or graveyard is often referred to as a "memorial garden," and a person does not "die" but "passes away"). In the last 60 years Hollywood has produced numerous cowboy shoot-outs, war scenes, mystery thrillers, gangster films, and adventure stories. In all these movies, death occurs during a dramatic moment. On the other hand, there have been virtually no movies of the slow death of a terminal patient, or the distintegration of the personality during senility. Apparently, there are few people who would be willing to attend such a viewing. Our society prefers to remain removed from the more normal occurrences of death, protected from any direct association with one of its most common experiences.[2]

However, a recent survey conducted by the National Opinion Research Center at the University of Chicago revealed that education (socioeconomic status is included within this context) and age, not sex or race, were the primary factors that affect one's perceptions and attitudes towards death. For example, there was a definite positive correlation between acquired formal education and planning for death (wills, life insurance, cemetary lots).[3]

Although men and women may make certain preparations for their eventual demise, there still exists a definite feeling of hostility towards death. As far as can be discerned, the human being is the only animal who consciously knows that one day he will die. Some social scientists believe that the fear of death is universal, and that no one is ever really free of it. Perhaps death's certainty (only the time, place, and staging are unknown) has caused Americans to cope by using mechanisms such as avoidance, denial, and repudiation.[4]

Factors Affecting Coping Techniques

Jeffers and Verwoerdt affirm that seven factors are critical in determining the type of coping techniques that an individual can use when facing death:

1) chronological age and distance from death;
2) physical and mental health;
3) various frames of reference such as religious orientation, socioeconomic and occupational status;
4) community attitudes;
5) family and personal experiences relating to death;
6) attitudes of people within the immediate environment;
7) the individual's psychological maturity and integrity.[5]

The Dying Process

Many books and articles have been written about the various stages that are associated with dying.

Kubler-Ross believes that denial, anger, bargaining, the organizing and completing of unfinished business, depression (reduction of interests, mourning of past losses, silently passing through preparatory grief), and acceptance (if the patient has been permitted to grieve and the family has acknowledged this total process, he will then be able to die in peace) are necessary stages of death and dying.[6]

Weisman postulates that death from terminal old age consists of the following phases: 1) repudiation of getting older, 2) denial of the extensions of aging, 3) denial of irreversible decline, 4) impaired autonomy, 5) a yielding of control and counter control, and 6) cessation of life.[7]

Attitudes of Professionals and Institutions Towards Death

Because most people feel that terminal old age is only a pause before life's cessation, the death of an old person in a hospital can be regarded in an almost casual way. Many elderly confused people are placed in an institution where they cope by renunciation (loss of choice and control), capitulation (acceptance of a standardized environment in which individuality is transformed into uniformity), nullification (loss of personal identity), and/or resolution. (A strategic equilibrium is achieved between control and counter-control. Although choice and control may be relinquished, there is an attempt on the part of the patient to preserve his social worth).[7]

Kubler-Ross states that our old age homes and nursing homes are a sad reflection of our lack of appreciation for our elders. Despite the fact that some retirement centers may have swimming pools and card rooms, she feels that we deprive our elderly of a chance to serve—an opportunity to offer the wisdom, experience, and skills that they have acquired over a lifetime. She also believes that if this right to serve others is denied, most older people may wish to die simply because life is not worth living. Kubler-Ross suggests that nursing homes and retirement centers should integrate their activities with children's programs, such as in day-care centers, where the elderly can be given an opportunity to help.[6]

In the review of a case history of a terminally ill patient, a team of professionals consisting of a physician, a psychiatrist, a minister, and a social psychologist agreed that in the area of death and dying most health care professionals impose emotional isolation upon the dying person, treat the dying person in a routine manner, and treat the patient as if he were an irresponsible child who cannot cope with his situation on an adult level; in other words, most helping professionals are unable to communicate to the patient and respond to his immediate needs and interests in an appropriate and adequate manner.[1] It is tragic, indeed, that with so little time left the dying patient is often robbed of the very meaning of life—consciousness, self-control, and decision making.[8]

Social Death: A Consequence of Institutional Attitudes

The concept of social death begins when the institution, accepting the impending death of the patient, loses its concern for the dying individual as a person and starts to treat him as if he were already dead. David Sudnow tells of two incidents that demonstrate this attitude. While at a 140-bed hospital (short-term general type, devoted to the care of acute illness, and operated to meet the needs of the indigent) he observed a nurse who spent several minutes trying to close the eyes of a dying female patient. When asked why she did this, the nurse replied that the lids were more difficult to close after death as the muscles and skin become stiff, and that this made for greater efficiency for ward personnel to prepare the body.

In another incident Sudnow observed that newly admitted patients who were near death (low blood pressure, erratic heart beats, nonpalpable pulse) were frequently left on the litter on which they had arrived and wheeled to a supply room or laboratory. Staff explained that this was necessary as it meant that a clean bed did not have to be used.

This investigator also noticed that as death approached, the attention shifted from a concern about life (possible comforts) and the administration of medically prescribed treatment to activities that involved the timing of events of biological death (ie, vital signs). Most patients in this particular hospital died unattended in a coma. Patients in this condition were considered to be unconscious. Thus, personnel talked freely in the patient's presence as if he were not there.[9]

Where People Die

Until the 20th century, most families cared for the sick and dying at home. With the advent of greater scientific and technical knowledge there has been a definite shift away from the home towards institutional care. In 1949, 49.5% of the population of this country died in institutions (convalescent and nursing homes, hospitals, hospital departments within institutions, and other types of domiciliary institutions). By 1958, 60.9% of all deaths occurred in institutions. The number of people who have died in institutional settings has been rising on an average of better then 1% annually during that time period.

A number of other nations have outdistanced us in the average person's life expectancy. Life expectancy in this country now appears to have reached a plateau at just above 70 years. However, in Australia, Denmark, the Netherlands, New Zealand, Norway, and Sweden the life expectancy may be as much as two or three years higher than comparable figures for the United States.* These statistics indicate that our total health care delivery system and life style should be improved.[10]

Our society's changing family structure (loss of the extended family) has also contributed to an increase of mortalities within the hospital or nursing home. Deaths now occur in settings that are removed from children and young adults. Instead of the warmth and support that is needed at this crucial time, most dying patients experience isolation, rejection, and loneliness.

New Programs on Death and Dying

Health care institutions, local Y's, adult centers, high schools, and colleges are offering many sensitivity courses on death and dying. Television specials that deal with the subject have contributed to an increasing awareness that death is a part of the life cycle.

The hospice concept, patterned on programs in Great Britain, is emerging in several areas of America. One of these in New Haven, Connecticut is now providing care for the terminally ill patient of any age who wants to remain at home as long as possible. The service, free to patients through funding by the National Cancer Institute, offers professionals and trained volunteers to provide care in the home. Emphasis is placed on pain control and helping the family deal with their feelings as well as with patient's. Hospice workers also offer support to grieving families after the patient has died.[11]

Occupational Therapy and the Dying Patient

Kubler-Ross tells us that one can communicate with the senile terminal patient through touch, love, and excellent nursing care.[6] Care to the dying includes involving them in life-process situations (decision making, awareness of the environment, continuing

United Nations Demographic Year Book, 1967, 562-583.

meaningful therapeutic treatments) until the end. The therapist can also assist the client, family, or staff in their adjustment to the dying process and meet the client's needs through active listening and support. Acknowledging and recognizing who these people are and what they have to say in their last moments is just as much a treatment as exercising an arm.[12]

By dealing with death and dying, the geriatric specialist has an opportunity to develop a deeper insight and understanding of his own life and death. No professional should ever feel that it is worthless to stroke the brow or wipe the sweat off the face of a dying elderly patient. The mature therapist realizes that life is as important at its end as it is in its beginning. The continuum of life is an experience that each one of us shares.

8

The Occupational Therapist as Consultant and Private Practitioner

---

Standards and Requirements

Although there have been a number of occupational therapy definitions, certain concepts have remained basic. Namely, occupational therapy, a professional service requested by a physician, is concerned with the improvement of impaired individuals' functioning levels. This includes the physical/psychosocial/cognitive dynamics of the client and is accomplished by means of assessment and treatment that utilizes purposeful activities and multi-modalities.[1]

In long term care the geriatric occupational therapist may work in several specialties—as a consultant, as an employee of an institution, and/or as a private practitioner. Each one of these categories has different functions as delineated by various funding and accrediting agencies.

Consultancy is an indirect service that involves the consultant's transmission of his professional knowledge and skill to solve problems (existing and potential). The consultant functions in an advisory capacity with no direct authority or responsibility for executing plans or programs. The consultee has the option of accepting or rejecting the consultant's suggestions.

In addition, the consultant can be involved in evaluating, identifying, and analyzing problem areas—instructing staff in therapeutic techniques and skills, assessing the patient's level of function, and determining appropriate rehabilitative programs and activities.

In nursing homes, many occupational therapists act as consultants to activities leaders (directors). According to Federal Regulations there are a number of patient activities requirements and

109

standards: "Provision is made for purposeful activities which are suited to the needs and interests of patients."* These regulations also designate that:

1) an individual be in charge of patient activities;

2) this individual be either experienced or in the process of training in directing group activities or be receiving consultation from a qualified group activity leader;

3) community, social, and recreational opportunities be used to their fullest extent by the activity leader;

4) patients be encouraged (never forced) to participate in these activities;

5) suitable activities be provided for those patients who are unable to leave their rooms;

6) patients who are able and who wish to attend religious services be assisted to those activities by activity personnel.

These patient activities regulations are similar for skilled nursing and intermediate care facilities.

The *Federal Register* defines consultancy in this way:

If the facility does not employ a qualified professional person to render a specific service to be provided by the facility, there are arrangements for such a service through a written agreement with an outside resource—a person or agency that will render direct service to patients or act as a consultant. The responsibilities, functions, and objectives, and the terms of agreement, including financial arrangements and charges, of each such outside resource are delineated in writing and signed by an authorized representative of the facility and the person or the agency providing the service. The agreement specifies that the facility retains professional and administrative responsibility for the services rendered. The financial arrangements provide that the outside resource bill the facility for covered services (either Part A or B for Medicare beneficiaries) rendered directly to the patient, and that receipt of payment from the program(s) to the facility for the services discharges the liability of the beneficiary or any other person to pay for the services. The outside resource, when acting as a consultant, apprises the administrator of recommendations, plans for implementation, and continuing assessment through dated, signed

Federal Health Insurance for the Aged. Conditions of Participation: Extended Care Facilities. (Title 20, Chapter 3, Part 405.1131), February, 1970.

reports, which are retained by the administrator for follow-up action and evaluation of performance.†

The presence of a qualified occupational therapy consultant does not convert an activity program into an occupational therapy service. To achieve this, individual (direct) patient treatment must be rendered by a registered occupational therapist. According to Federal Regulations 504.1126(d) for extended care facilities (Title 20, Chapter III, Feb, 1970) occupational therapy, part of restorative services, is prescribed by a physician who determines the objectives, modality, and frequency of therapy. The therapist can assist the physician in the evaluation of the patient's functioning level (by means of diagnostic and prognostic tests). Patient care plans are a result of collaborative efforts between medical and nursing staff. The therapist can advise the administrator as to the purchase, storage, rental, and maintenance of equipment and supplies. Regulations are very similar for skilled nursing and intermediate care facilities.

Private practice is also a direct service that involves the occupational therapist as a provider of individual treatment. The therapist's responsibilities include evaluating the patient's level of function, planning and implementing appropriate treatment, and documenting patient progress.

The federal government is not the only determiner of health care standards; each state also sets standards, and several special organizations such as the Commission for Accreditation of Rehabilitation Facilities (CARF) and the Joint Commission on Accreditation of Hospitals (JCAH) require an adherence to regulations. JCAH is responsible for accrediting long term care facilities, psychiatric facilities, services for mental retardation, ambulatory health care, and services to developmentally disabled persons. In a recent statement this commission emphasized that the quality of patient care is the central objective of its entire process of accreditation.[2] Since standards and regulations directly affect service, each therapist should be knowledgeable about his state's and facility's requirements.

---

†*Skilled Nursing Facilities.* The Federal Register. *Standards for Participation in Medicare and Medicaid Programs. Vol 39, No 10, (405.1121), January 17, 1974.*

Consultancy And Private Practice Settings

Consultants and private practitioners may serve in a number of settings: nursing homes, hospitals, day care centers, residential halls, community mental health centers, and individual homes.

Generally, most consultants practice in long term care institutions (nursing homes, infirmaries sometimes referred to as medical centers). These institutions are located within homes for the aged or retirement communities, chronic disease hospitals (terminal care homes), mental hospitals, veteran administration hospitals, and other specialty hospitals.[3]

Since most occupational therapy consultancies occur in nursing homes, a brief description of nursing home categories is helpful:

Proprietary (Commercial) Facilities—This refers to private profit-making nursing homes.

Extended Care Facilities—Derived from Medicare legislation, these facilities are an extension of hospital care with a probability of discharge.

Skilled Nursing Care Facilities—This term, derived from Medicaid, refers to long term, unlimited nursing care. There is no requirement of previous hospitalization. Funding is provided by a federal-state cost sharing program.

Intermediate Care Facilities—Designed to give personal care, simple medical care, and intermittent nursing care, intermediate care facilities are funded through Medicaid.[4]

Reimbursement

Most consultancy services are reimbursed through third party payers—Blue Cross and Blue Shield, Medicare, Medicaid, and commercial insurance companies. The individual that receives the service is termed *first party;* the institution or individual performing the service is the *second party;* and the organization paying for it is the *third party.*

Appropriate documentation based on insurance requirements is essential. For example, diversional treatment will not be reimbursed by third party payers.[1] Requirements for evaluations and progress notes will be detailed in Chapter 10.

Contacting Prospective Employers

First one needs to know the exact location of available nursing homes. This can be achieved by writing to the local state nursing home association and asking for a list of accredited homes or by looking in the yellow pages of the telephone book. Job opportunities are advertised in professional journals and commercial newspapers. Another method is to contact private professional employment agencies.

The therapist who canvasses by telephone or mail should include his education and work experience. But, most important, he should state what he can offer in the way of therapeutic services.

An interview where the administrator and prospective consultant have an opportunity to evaluate each other and to discuss related duties and responsibilities is essential. Once a verbal agreement is reached, a written contract should be initiated which specifically delineates the following:

1) duties of the occupational therapist as consultant (including specific consultancy requirements to the activity program leader);

2) the occupational therapist's direct responsibilities to the patient (eg, evaluating, treatment planning, record keeping);

3) specific responsibilities to other agency sources (administrative, nursing, dietary);

4) required frequency of consultation and fee schedule.

There should also be a statement concerning termination of services. Usually 30 days written notification of intent to terminate on the behalf of both parties is sufficient.

This document should be signed and dated by the therapist and nursing home administrator.

Interviews

There are many ways in which an individual can acquire knowledge. Books, journals, and closed circuit television are some examples. The verbal transmission of past experiences is an older, yet meaningful and successful way to learn.

The following interviews of two therapists who work as consultants and private practitioners detail their thoughts and concerns regarding Occupational Therapy. In the case of these and other interviews, the interviewees' ideas are individual and are not necessarily reflective of the institutions that they may serve.

Interview with Leba Grodinsky, OTR**

Lewis: What first made you decide to become involved in private practice?

Grodinsky: I had retired for 15 years and a friend of mine encouraged me to get back into the field, suggesting a partnership in a private practice of Occupational Therapy. Initially, we operated out of her house and a local church. I have always liked the flexibility and freedom that this type of practice affords.

Lewis: What do you consider to be the most important aspect of your work?

Grodinsky: The most important aspect is to convince the staff, other professionals, the client and family members of the rehabilitation to which I have a firm commitment— which is the obligation to allow the client to live his life at 100% of his capabilities.

Lewis: Are your contracts of a verbal or written nature?

Grodinsky: The contracts that I use are written, with a complete job description of my duties.

Lewis: What types of settings have you worked in as a private practitioner?

Grodinsky: I have helped develop an outpatient rehabilitation program in a private hospital and have worked in a variety of nursing homes and family settings.

Lewis: Has the advent of Medicare affected your practice?

Grodinsky: Yes, it has helped to pay for occupational therapy rehabilitation programs. Formerly, many clients would not have been able to afford and receive this type of service. In fact, I believe it has made it possible for a larger number of occupational therapists to become involved in nursing home consultancy.

Lewis: Would you discuss a specific case history in which an elderly person was helped by your service?

**Printed with permission by Mrs. Leba Grodinsky, OTR, private practitioner.*

Grodinsky: Mrs. K, a 78-year-old Caucasian widow, nursed her husband through a series of mental illnesses in their home. During her marriage she assumed a variety of duties beyond the role of homemaker (ie, roofer, painter, gardener, and carpenter). She was also a skilled painter of miniature art. Mrs. K lived alone for many years until her stroke.

On her first admission to the nursing home she was diagnosed as a right CVA with a residual left hemiplegia. She was dependent for all self-care except for feeding and was extremely depressed.

She became involved in an occupational therapy and physical therapy rehabilitation program. Mrs. K's occupational therapy treatment goals were 1) to attain greater independence in self-care, 2) to improve balance in sitting and standing, and 3) to increase motivation towards greater socialization by including her in a hemiplegia exercise and discussion group. Mrs. K's personal goal was to be discharged as soon as possible to her own home. She was adamant about this, and despite the fact that the rehabilitation team advised her not to leave at that time, she returned to her home in the care of her niece. Initially, Mrs. K's niece had agreed to accept this responsibility for a brief period. Upon discharge she needed assistance in standing, walking, and self-care.

This home arrangement did not work well, and she returned to the nursing home within two months. On her second admission she had frequent falls in her attempts to be as independent as possible.

At this time she began daily treatment in an OT program using a combination of sensorimotor treatment techniques, stressing weight bearing on upper and lower extremities, weight shifting, and balance reactions in movement patterns following a developmental sequence. She has since progressed to the point (within one year) where she can walk independently with a "quad cane," and is totally independent in self-care. There have been no further incidents of falls.

Mrs. K is now resuming some of her former skills (for instance, painting miniatures) and enjoys socializing with peers and staff.

Lewis: What advice would you offer a novice occupational therapist coming into the field of private practice?

Grodkinsky: One should assume the duties of consultant carefully. It is essential to listen closely to others (the client, the family, the nursing home administrator, nursing staff, etc) to hear what they are saying. The acquisition of new knowledge and a genuine interest in people is also important. It is necessary to feel comfortable and be able to relate well, especially when working with geriatric clients. Finally, one should be aware and appreciate the fact that the older client has had a life style that is very different from that of the present generation.

Interview with Cindy Brillman, OTR‡

Lewis: What first made you decide to become involved in occupational therapy private practice and consultancy?

Brillman: After I graduated from college, I applied for several jobs. However, I wasn't excited about filling an "ordinary" staff position as I like challenge. I then wrote a cover letter explaining the role of occupational therapy to many nursing homes in the area. I received responses from several of these nursing homes. One of the homes wanted to initiate an occupational therapy physical dysfunction department. This was my first job. It was also the first occupational therapy physical dysfunction department in a nursing home in Pennsylvania. I worked from 9:00 A.M. to 4:30 P.M. during the week. I then began to apply for part-time occupational therapy positions in other nursing homes. Later, I started to work at night, especially at the dinner hour.

‡*Printed with permission by Mrs. Cindy Brillman, OTR, consultant and private practitioner.*

116

Eventually, I had to give up my full-time job because my private practice grew so large.

Lewis: What is the most important aspect of your job?

Brillman: The most important aspect is to be able to convey to the nursing home personnel the importance and function of occupational therapy. To do this one has to be able to explain what occupational therapy is to people on various intellectual levels.

Lewis: Would you describe your work responsibilities?

Brillman: Specific occupational therapy services I provide include *evaluation and re-evaluation* of the following: upper extremity function, perception, cognition, self-care, orthotic, prosthetic, cardiac, and newly blind/partially sighted; *activities involving kinetic treatment programs* such as range of motion, facilitation, sensation, muscle re-education, endurance, strengthening, dexterity, sitting balance and tolerance, and standing balance and tolerance; and *specific areas of training such as* perception, sensation, self-care, joint protection, work simplification, transfers and wheel chair mobility, and home instruction where necessary. Much of my work involves inservices to auxiliary personnel. Other program involvement includes reality orientation, remotivation, and movement therapy. The occupational therapist also often functions as a consultant to the nursing home's activity personnel.

When one is working for himself/herself, other personal responsibilities are required such as paying one's withholding tax and meeting one's social security needs, providing one's own benefits (hospitalization, malpractice insurance, accident insurance, pension plan), billing the nursing home, buying equipment for the patient as well as for the therapist, and justifying one's treatment to Medicare.

Lewis: Are your contracts of a verbal or written nature?

Brillman: My contracts are written. They are a very specific description as to what the nursing home requires of me and what I require of them. My contracts include the exact hours that I work, my specific role, when and how I get paid, and malpractice responsibilities of the nursing home (even though I have my own).

Lewis: Would you clarify the differences between consultancy and private practice?

Brillman: Medicare's definition of consultant is one who acts as an adviser. A consultant does not treat patients. One's responsibilities are to make suggestions to the nursing home in the ways that they can improve their services which apply to occupational therapy. However, there is a misnomer concerning the definition of consultant among some nursing homes. Although a therapist may be treating patients, the nursing home may call the therapist a consultant because she/he works part-time.

Private practice means "being in business for yourself." You are able to treat patients and get reimbursed for your services by Medicare.

Lewis: What types of notes does Medicare require?

Brillman: Medicare requires one to always show progress/lack of progress and justification for continued treatment. Medicare is not interested in the concept of maintenance but focuses upon improving the client's condition. In writing notes one must be very specific in describing the client's level of function.

Lewis: What prompted you to become initially involved in writing occupational therapy coverage proposals for Blue Cross (Pennsylvania)?

Brillman: I wasn't receiving occupational therapy coverage in nursing homes which use Blue Cross as an intermediary (even though the Medicare regulations specifically stated and outlined Occupational Therapy coverage).

Lewis: What type of process was necessary in order to obtain this coverage?

Brillman: The entire process took one full year. Initially I contacted a Blue Cross official who was knowledgeable about occupational therapy coverage. Next, I wrote a proposal stating the role of occupational therapy as well as the justification for occupational therapy in a nursing home as provided by a private practitioner. Later, I met many Blue Cross officials as well as physicians employed by Blue Cross. At these meetings I had to justify the level of care given by an occupational therapist in private practice.

Lewis: Would you discuss a specific case history in which an elderly individual was helped by your service?

Brillman: Mrs. X, a 72-year-old Caucasian widow who lived alone in an apartment, had multiple diagnoses on admission to the nursing home. These included a left CVA (flaccid right upper and lower extremities), left wrist drop due to previous injury, cardiovascular disease (high blood pressure), legally blind, and rheumatoid arthritis (with minimal physical deformities).

The initial occupational therapy evaluation indicated 1) dependence in all areas of ADL (dressing, eating, personal hygiene), 2) strength in left upper extremity was poor +, 3) transfers required maximal assistance, and 4) standing balance and tolerance was poor.

The occupational therapy goals and treatment methods included the following.

1) Basic ADL program was initiated (upper extremity dressing and personal hygiene were introduced as well as basic eating and cutting techniques). Adaptive equipment was utilized.

2) Techniques to improve left upper extremity strengthening were initiated.

3) Standing tolerance and balance exercises were introduced.

4) Facilitation techniques were administered at every session.

5) Basic transfer techniques (from bed to chair, chair to toilet) to improve independence were initiated.

Mrs. X responded well to facilitation and in three months she was able to perform all upper extremity dressing and personal hygiene techniques. Her standing balance and tolerance had also improved. She could independently transfer to toilet and in and out of bed. She was also able to independently feed herself as well as cut her food and manage her tray. Mrs. X's left upper extremity strength had greatly improved and her right upper extremity was now functional.

New occupational therapy goals were set. These included improving independence by introducing two additional treatment programs—1) lower extremity dressing and personal hygiene, and 2) transfers in and out of the tub.

After a period of one and a half months these goals were accomplished. Plans for discharge were then initiated, and new goals were set involving homemaking skills.

By six months Mrs. X was discharged to her home. Her rehabilitation was so complete that at the time of her discharge she was able to resume independent living in her own apartment.

Lewis: What advice would you offer a novice occupational therapist coming into the field of consultancy/private practice?

Brillman: First, one should know Medicare and her/his state regulations. Next, one should be prepared to be able to explain to involved personnel an "on the spot" explanation of the role of occupational therapy as well as the justification for occupational therapy. Finally, one should be able to be flexible and patient.

Concluding Remarks

There is little doubt that consultancy, presently in a nascent state, will continue to grow as our elderly population increases. Flexibility and a desire and ability to problem solve are key factors to success in this area of specialization.

Private practice and consultancy offer a number of options and management possibilities: incorporation, partnership, and sole ownership. As a consultant, the therapist has unique opportunities to develop self-reliance, independence, and expertise.

9

Community Occupational Therapy Programs

Ninety-five percent of this country's elders live in their community.[1] Of this group it is estimated that one out of every seven requires some type of supportive service in order to maintain independent living.[2] As our aging population grows, one can assume that there will be an ever increasing need to provide programs that enable older persons to live in their own residences as long as possible.

Community-Oriented Programs

There are a variety of health care programs (eg, geriatric day hospitals, adult day treatment centers, community mental health centers, programs to prevent institutionalization, neighborhood center programs, and visiting nurse associations and home health care agencies) offering supportive approaches that help the client maintain himself within his community.

Federal regulations, under titles 18 (Part B) and 19 of the Social Security Act, have made public funding of geriatric day hospital and day care programs possible.

According to Federal Guidelines, day care is defined as a program of services that provide health care in an ambulatory setting for adults who do not need 24-hour institutional care, but due to mental and physical dysfunction, are not able to cope with full-time independent living.*

Kiernat cautions that one should discern the differences between senior centers or day centers for older people that provide

Guidelines and definitions for day care services to be carried out in experiments and demonstrations under P.L. 92-603, Section 222(b), Washington DC, June 1974.

recreational and social programs and day hospitals and day care services that provide therapeutic programs in a protective environmental setting for impaired elders. In the day hospital/day care setting older clients are transported from their homes to a center (maybe housed in a nursing home, hospital, or extended care facility) that provides access to medical, nursing, and allied therapies available within the institution.[3]

Day Hospitals

At the Maimonides Day Hospital in Montreal, Quebec, Canada, the primary goal is to delay or prevent institutionalization. The focus is upon maintenance, rehabilitation, and supervisory services. The occupational therapist's role is divided into several areas: 1) initial individual assessments and periodic reassessments, 2) supervising and monitoring activities programs, 3) individual and small group treatment sessions, 4) home visits, and 5) cooperation with staff in maintaining a therapeutic milieu.[4]

The Day Hospital at the Burke Rehabilitation Center in White Plains, New York provides the following rehabilitative treatment services: medical, dietary and nutritional counseling, health education, nursing, personal care, occupational therapy, speech therapy, physical therapy, activities therapy, social services, and transportation. The program is designed to provide two levels of treatment: 1) intensive (short-term individual sessions) and 2) intermediate (long-term group-oriented activities). In the intensive level program, occupational therapists are responsible for providing functional exercises and activities, home making, perceptual training, activities of daily living, opportunities to improve communication and socialization skills, and home assessments and home care plans. The intermediate level program includes organized group activities that are designed to maintain residual function as well as provide social and mental stimulation.[5] Programming at this center was funded initially by a grant from the Administration on Aging (HEW).

Adult Day Treatment Centers

The Adult Day Treatment Center of Beverly Hills, California, is a private psychiatric facility that provides a program which promotes the therapeutic use of activities to improve the patient's optimum level of functioning. The modalities used to accomplish this include art therapy; psychodrama; dance therapy; discussion of world events; food and nutrition counseling; physical re-education; group psychotherapy, resocialization techniques; the use of games to provide appropriate communication outlets and improve skills (eg, bridge, dominoes, scrabble); and community field trips (eg, art galleries, museums, community centers, shopping trips, and restaurant outings). The occupational therapist's responsibilities include the following:

1) administering individual patient assessments, (eg, physical strength, range of motion, activities of daily living, eye-hand coordination, orientation as to time, place, person and personal interest profile — with emphasis upon intake and history, if possible, from an interested family member);
2) to provide instruction in and the development of hobbies as a means to rebuild and increase ego-strength;
3) to provide appropriate opportunities for ventilating feelings and expressing anger and hostility by means of appropriate therapeutic projects;
4) to provide opportunities to reclaim and strengthen old skills (eg, decision making, organizing, planning, communication, and interaction with others) through activities such as cooking, woodworking, needle crafts, and self-care;
5) to provide appropriate physical and self-care programs (eg, instruction in activities of daily living, muscle strengthening exercises).[6]

The need for adult day care will certainly increase as our aging population continues to expand.

Community Mental Health Care Centers

Occupational therapists are beginning to fulfill major roles in the area of providing innovative and meaningful programs for geriatric clients in community mental health centers. An example of such a program is the Outreach Activity Group of District V Mental Health Center of the North Central Florida Community Mental Health Center. The University of Florida's Department of Occupational Therapy was responsible for helping to implement, collaborate, and participate in this therapeutic group. The program was conducted in an outlying high school and transportation was provided by a local church. The client population consisted of former hospitalized elderly patients who were living in isolated rural areas. Goals for the Outreach Activity Group consisted of developing mutual trust and respect among members, promoting and supporting feelings of dignity and self-worth, maintaining and promoting physical capabilities, increasing awareness of community resources, encouraging self-expression on verbal and nonverbal levels, providing new interest and constructive use of leisure time, encouraging interpersonal interactions, increasing opportunities for reality testing, and providing cognitive-perceptual motor stimulation.

Modalities within the program format included discussion (involving stories, recipes, personal and group concerns, local history and cultural heritage), eating, singing, movement and exercise, participation in crafts, groups and/or team games, group awareness techniques, and tactile stimulation (eg, back massage, patting, touching oneself. and others).[7] This type of creative and purposeful program provides elderly people who might be subject to rehospitalization with opportunities to reinforce and maintain independence.

Programs to Prevent Institutionalization

Intervention programs designed to prevent institutional placement are of paramount importance. Not only will these help decrease bed demand, they will also provide the older person with a renewed opportunity to remain in the community. The Geriatric Community Evaluation and Treatment Service Team at the Norristown State Hospital (Norristown, Pennsylvania) exemplified this type of service.

The service offered personalized and preventive psychiatric, medical, and social attention to distressed elders. This mobile team, consisting of three geropsychiatrists, three social workers, one liaison visiting nurse, one occupational therapy consultant, one therapeutic recreational consultant, and two secretaries, handled referrals to the hospital of disturbed older adults (65+).

The approach, one of immediate and flexible interaction, permitted problem solving at the older person's place of residence.

Three basic tenets of the service involved 1) the diagnosis and treatment of the presenting problem, 2) prevention and/or resolution of the impending family or residential staff crises which had led to the original referral, and 3) introduction of social and psychiatric safeguards to ensure the client's long-term success in the community. In over 8½ years of existence, the service team had evaluated some 1,438 troubled elderly people and consulted with 77 nursing or retirement homes. In that time, only 222 clients required admission to the hospital.[8] During this time the occupational therapist was primarily responsible for activities program consultancy to nursing homes, residential centers, and boarding homes that utilized the service. The success of such a service ensures the elderly client that every possible option or alternative to prevent institutional placement will be examined.

Neighborhood Center Programs

The support of the Madison (Wisconsin) Neighborhood Center for the Independent Living Project for the elderly (presently entitled Services to Maintain Independent Living for the Elderly) demonstrates that a community based program can indeed be essential in helping an older person live a satisfactory and independent life within his neighborhood.

Staff consisted of a part-time occupational therapy consultant, a half-time administrative assistant, and a half-time bus driver. The program concerned itself with adult education, home consultation, and transportation. These services were offered to older persons without any fee.

Adult education classes, consisting of five courses—Self-care for the Person Confined to a Wheelchair, Independent Living Techniques for the One-handed Individual, Methods in Solving the Problems of Daily Living for the Arthritic Client, Everyday Helps for the Visually Handicapped, and Daily Independent Living for the Cardiac, provided topical information that was beneficial in helping elders maintain themselves in their community. Other general meetings (such as consumer protection, special telephone services for older adults, social security information, tax form preparation, and information on community services available to elders in the community) were scheduled for the entire elderly population.

Home consultation by an occupational therapy consultant was another important aspect of the program. Consulting responsibilities included home evaluations, recommendations for improving the home environment (eg, shower seats, grab bars, raised toilet seats, sliding kitchen shelves) and safety, and/or appropriate referrals to other agencies and services (ie, Meals on Wheels, Visiting Nurse, and Home Maker Home Health Aids).

Transportation was the third component of this project. The Neighborhood House bus was used to take older people on regularly scheduled trips to supermarkets and shopping centers. Clients could also request transportation to dental and doctor's appointments or any other type of essential visit.[9] Occupational therapists working in this type of setting can reach a large number of older citizens.

Home Health Care Agencies

Home health care, such as provided by a visiting nurse association or a private agency, permits citizens to receive health care in the privacy of their own home. According to Medicare, occupational therapy coverage is defined as a

...medically prescribed treatment concerned with improving or restoring functions which have been impaired by illness or injury or, where function has been permanently lost or reduced by illness or injury, to improve the individual's ability to perform those tasks required for independent functioning.†

Therapy may include a number of functions:

1. evaluation and re-evaluation of the patient's level of functioning by the administration of diagnostic and prognostic tests;
2. selection and teaching of task-oriented therapeutic activities designed to restore physical function;
3. planning, implementing, and supervising of individualized therapeutic activity programs which are part of an overall "active treatment" program for a patient with a diagnosed psychiatric illness;
4. planning and implementing therapeutic tasks and activities to restore sensory-integrative functioning;

†*Home Health Agency Manual Revision. US Department of Health, Education and Welfare, No 72, November 1975, 205.d.*

126

5. teaching compensatory techniques to improve independent functioning in activities of daily living;
6. designing, fabricating, and fitting orthotic and self-help devices;
7. vocational and prevocational assessment and training.

Medicare coverage (205.2B) involves specific requirements:
1) that the service be *prescribed* by a physician;
2) that it be *performed* by a qualified occupational therapist or by a qualified occupational therapy assistant under the general supervision of a qualified occupational therapist (however, only a qualified occupational therapist can evaluate the patient's level of function and determine an appropriate treatment plan);
3) that the therapy is *reasonable* and *necessary* (interpreted to mean only where an expectation exists that the service will result in significant practical improvement of the individual's level of function within a reasonable period of time).

It is important to note that while coverage is provided for designing a maintenance program and for making infrequent and periodic evaluation of its effectiveness, the services of an occupational therapist or an occupational therapy assistant are not covered for payment for carrying out such a program.

At present Medicare coverage for occupational therapy is inadequate. Specifically section 1814 [a] [2] [D] and section 1835 [a] [2] [A] of Title XVIII of the Social Security Act omit occupational therapy as a single outpatient service. This means that as a condition for payment for home health services, a physician must certify that the patient needs home health services in the form of skilled nursing care or that physical or speech therapy must be a required service (prerequisite) that accompanies occupational therapy. The National Office of the American Occupational Therapy Association has been very active in trying to have this part of the Social Security Act amended so that coverage of occupational therapy as a single outpatient service will become a reality.

Statistics show that within a nine year period, home health agencies in the United States have grown from 1,163 to approximately 2,300 agencies.** It would appear that this trend towards

**Day Care Services. Washington DC, Office of Policy, Planning and Evaluation, Medical Services Administration, Social and Rehabilitation Service, US Department of Health, Education and Welfare, 1972.*

increasing home health care will continue as this type of service provides alternatives to institutional care. The number of practicing occupational therapists in the field of home health care has also been increasing rapidly.

Interviews

The following interviews by two therapists working in the community (occupational therapy consultancy in a home health care agency and transitional community residential care) demonstrate the effectiveness of occupational therapy in this important area of specialization.

Interview with Ruth Levine, M.Ed., OTR‡

Lewis: What first made you decide to become involved in community occupational therapy programs and services?

Levine: Originally I wanted to work with a drug addiction population, but my clinical field work coordinator teacher, Clare Spackman, suggested that I look into a job at the Community Nursing Service of Philadelphia. When I graduated from college in 1969, occupational therapists were rarely involved in community service; therefore, I was not aware that this was a viable alternative to inpatient clinical work. The person who interviewed me at Community Nursing Service was eager to hire an occupational therapist and supported some of the ideas that I discussed with her.

Lewis: What do you consider to be the most important personality traits for therapists who do home care work?

Levine: Basically, there is a need for a pragmatic individual who is flexible and can problem solve in a variety of different social structures. He or she must be a generalist with good group dynamic skills. The goal of the home care agency team is to teach other family members or caretakers to carry out treatment programs and care for the client. Thus, technical programs must be simplified so that

‡*Printed with permission of Ruth Levine, M.Ed., O.T.R., Director of Community Occupational Therapy Consultants, Director of Occupational Therapy Community Education at Temple University, Philadelphia, Pa.*

family members can render daily treatment.

Lewis: Would you discuss a specific case history in which an elderly individual was helped by your service?

Levine: Mr. M. was a black, 67-year-old lower bilateral amputee with a right hemiplegia on his dominant side. He was aphasic and diabetic also. He lived with his wife in a public housing project. Mr. M. was referred to occupational therapy by a Public Health nurse who wanted to promote his dressing skills. Mr. M. was visited by the occupational therapist who found that his goal was not in the area of ADL, but rather to increase the functioning of his right upper extremity. The occupational therapist introduced exercises and a bilateral activity — a turkish knotted rug. Mr. M. worked religiously at his exercises and his rug which gradually became a total investment for him. Even on days when he felt very ill, Mr. M. reported that he was compelled to do a minimal amount of work on his rug. Treatment continued for six months. During this period he almost died twice, but he always managed to struggle through. Also during this time he and his wife shared momentos of their life together. The occupational therapist supported this interaction between husband and wife and assumed the role of active listener. One week after the rug was completed Mr. M. died. On the last occupational therapy visit Mrs. M. proudly displayed Mr. M.'s rug. This was the last activity that they had shared. Although saddened by Mr. M's death, she seemed able to accept this fact peacefully.

Lewis: Even though a client may be dying, should all attempts be made to continue treatment?

Levine: I personally believe they should. No therapist is skilled enough to determine the exact date of any person's death.

Lewis: What advice would you offer a novice occupational therapist coming into the field of home health care services?

Levine: Basically the person needs skills in both psychosocial and physical dysfunction occupational therapy. Primarily, one needs to know how to relate to the joys and tragedies of daily life and still love people. A final point is that the therapist must lead a balanced life so that he or she can develop an individual philosophy toward all aspects of life, including illness and dying as well as health and living.

Interview with Susan Chain Parker, OTR*

Lewis: What first made you decide to become involved in adult day care and transitional services?

Parker: Interest started when I worked in a large state hospital's admission's unit, and I became aware of the rapid rate of recidivism. This resulted in my realization of the need for a support system in the community for those being discharged from mental hospitals.

Lewis: What do you consider to be the most important aspect of your work?

Parker: I consider the responsibility for program development as the most important aspect of my work.

Lewis: What are your present responsibilities?

Parker: My responsibilities include program development for day treatment, program development for evening residency programs, supervision of social service aides who implement the programs, purchasing all needed materials for the programs, obtaining appropriate furnishings for the residences (houses and apartments), development of community resources (ie, nutrition programs, athletic programs, league of women voters, etc), coordinating billing of clients, and coordinating transportation schedules for programs.

Lewis: Would you discuss a specific case history in which an elderly individual was helped by your service?

Parker: Mr. X, a 76-year-old Caucasion divorced male, had his initial hospitalization at the age of 75. This hospitalization was a direct result of a suicide attempt (overdose of thyroid pills). Since his divorce of 30 years, Mr. X had resided alone and had provided his livelihood as a short order cook in New York City. Nine months prior to his psychiatric hospitalization, he suffered a stroke and went

*Printed with permission by Susan Chain Parker, O.T.R., Assistant Supervisor of the Transitional Residency Program, Delaware House, Burlington, New Jersey.

to live with his son in New Jersey on discharge. Mr. X was hospitalized at the state hospital for several months. However, placement was a problem since he could not return to his son's home. It was at this time that he was referred to Delaware House residential program. Mr. X was placed in a 24 hour supervised house. His presenting symptoms/behaviors were his impairment of memory, his irresponsibility, and periodic episodes of hallucinations predominately pertaining to religion.

The treatment goals set with Mr. X were as follows.

1) A graded approach to responsibility was provided by the residential staff.
2) A small notebook was encouraged to be used by Mr. X to help him remember duties, appointments, phone numbers, etc.
3) Alternative interests, such as editing and writing for the Delaware House newsletter, were encouraged in order to divert his religious preoccupation.

After two months Mr. X improved sufficiently to move to a more independent situation—an apartment with three other clients. The goals at this time were altered to meet his new needs. These included his learning to care for and to support his other roommates as well as his acquisition of increased independence (ie, budgeting, menu planning, sharing household chores, leisure time activities, etc).

Lewis: What advice would you offer a novice occupational therapist coming into the field of adult day care and transitional services?

Parker: The individual should learn to tap any and all community resources. One's personal life experiences should be varied and full. A person should make the most of any experience because one never knows how this information can be utilized at some future time. Flexibility and adaptability are the two key words.

Concluding Remarks

Community occupational therapy is rapidly expanding. Therapists specializing in this area have an opportunity to serve and acquaint the public with occupational therapy skills and knowledge. The clients, their needs, and enormous professional challenges await the interested and proficient geriatric practitioner. The demand for occupational therapy services in community health has never been greater.

10

Designing and Promoting Educational and Informative Experiences

Continuing Professional Education

Professional education can be enhanced by reading books, magazines, and journals that pertain to gerontology; discussing evaluations, procedures, treatment techniques, and methods with knowledgeable clinicians; observing geriatric programs; and attending courses, workshops, lectures, and seminars that are focused upon geriatrics.

Those practitioners who have accumulated expertise in geriatric occupational therapy should obligate themselves to share this knowledge with their fellow therapists. One way to accomplish this is by documenting successful programs and techniques. Another method is to involve a number of proficient geriatric specialists as leaders of organized workshops and seminars.

Professional Workshops and Seminars

This section is concerned with the organizational and administrative techniques that are needed to achieve a successful workshop or seminar (eg, committee structure and responsibilities, purposeful goals, appropriate content designed to meet the workshop's stated objectives, and assessment tools to evaluate the effectiveness of the workshop or seminar).

Committee Structure and Responsibilities

In initiating an educational experience it is essential to establish a committee headed by a coordinator(s) that will act to organize and distribute the workload. Once the goals and purposes have been collectively established by the committee, each member can then assume specific responsibilities: establishing content (specific topics); contacting presenters; designing the program and preparing flyers; arranging for the appropriate use of advertising media such as radio and professional journals; obtaining a locale that is accessible to public transportation and has adequate parking facilities; acquiring needed audiovisual devices such as a public address system, slide projectors, screens, movie projectors and audio-visual receivers; providing adequate luncheon arrangements (if the event is to be an all day experience); establishing a fee structure (an admission charge, sponsorship by an institution or organization, and/or procurement of a grant are ways that can be utilized to cover the cost); and developing an evaluation instrument that can be used to measure the audiences' assessment of the project.

The most important aspect to be concerned with is understanding the significant needs of practitioners and to then be responsive to these needs. In order to insure success, the seminar must contain meaningful and useful subject matter.

Content

What types of information do therapists and students seek? From this therapist's personal experience, the topics most often requested fall into the following categories: 1) *geriatric occupational therapy programs and treatment techniques,* 2) *documentation,* and 3) *staff development.*

Since treatment programs and techniques have already been examined, (Chapter 6 pp 61-100 and Chapter 9 pp 121-132 we shall turn our discussion to professional documentation.

Professional Documentation

Assessments—A General View

Assessment and/or evaluation of patient progress is an ongoing, essential aspect of documentation. Initial assessments are particularly important as they provide a baseline from which the effectiveness of treatment can be determined or measured. Periodic assessments are also important as they provide the therapist with continuous knowledge of the patient's problem areas and/or development. When treatment is terminated, the therapist should administer a final assessment of the patient's performance using the same evaluation instrument(s) throughout the entire treatment process.

Evaluation and/or assessment are problem solving tools for defining current needs or conditions, determining outcome, planning, and research. Evaluation is specifically necessary where there is a choice among alternatives in professional care-giving.

Tests used to evaluate patient performance vary considerably, generally in five areas.

1) *General purpose*—classify, describe, select, and/or predict.

2) *Degree of standardization*—norms are standardized distributions of scores by specified subjects that are based on extensive research with large representative samples of such subjects.

3) *Comprehensiveness of measurements*—eg, measures of extreme performance such as the best or least effective level of functioning, or typical performance.

4) *Administration methods*—eg, group or individual, time, ease, and specified skills spent in giving and scoring of the test(s).

5) *Degree of established validity and reliability.* Test validity involves three components—content, criterion-relatedness, and construct. Specifically, *content validity* is the systematic examination of the items contained within a test that are used to determine the effectiveness of the representative sample of behavior that is being measured. *Criterion-relatedness* involves predictable and concurrent measures. These are employed in diagnosing the existing status of the patient. *Construct validity* is the extent to which a test measures a theoretical trait. This type of validity may involve internal consistency or correlation with other tests (ie, a positive correlation with variables that are theoretically related) and the degree of obtrusiveness (the obviousness or nonobviousness of a test).[1]

The objectivity of a test is important: an assessment instrument should lend itself to administration and scoring without the results being affected by the personal judgment of the assessor.

Bloom discusses the factors that he considers essential areas of functioning for long term care clients. These could be adapted and used as assessment categories for most geriatric clients. They include six functions.

1) *Survival*—A basic but often overlooked factor.

2) *Physical functioning*—This involves physical health as viewed in the context and application to daily living.

3) *Mental functioning*—This includes intellectual ability, problem solving capabilities, orientation, and judgment.

4) *Affective functioning*—A basic concern in this area is how older persons emotionally respond to the problems of adapting and coping with life. This includes examining the pathological aspects of feeling states as well as measures of life satisfaction (degree of contentment, well-being, morale).

5) *Social and interpersonal functioning*—(some investigators may regard this area to be directly related to category three). This topic considers the degree that a client relates to significant social others on either a casual or sustained basis between family, friend, or acquaintance.

6) *Environmental functioning*—This area is concerned with how much a client influences his physical and social environment, and how he, in turn, is influenced by them.[1]

Lawton recognizes seven basic classes of behavior that can also serve as appropriate assessment areas of human functioning. These include life maintenance (eg, breathing), functional health (eg house-bound), perception-cognition (eg, short-term memory), physical self-maintenance (eg, grooming), instrumental self-maintenance (eg, financial management), effectance (eg, curiousity), and social role (eg, close contact.)[2]

If the data source is viewed as a continuum, then one end consists of the client's own responses as the source of information *(client data)*. Client data is obtained from situations in which the client is his own scribe (ie, paper and pencil tests of his own feelings or an interview process that may be structured, unstructured, or mixed).

At the opposite end of the continuum the observer's responses become the data *(observer data)*. This includes the observer's interpretations and judgments that are often based upon constructed group norms against which an individual client's responses are compared.

The obstrusiveness of the data collection procedure is another important factor. *Instrument data compilation* involves collecting information by means of a questionnaire form, various mechanical tests and devices, and simulated or artificial environments that act as an impetus for collecting information about the client. On the other hand, *non-reactive data collection* utilizes traces of client behavior that were not initially performed for purposes of measurement.[1]

Assessment—Specific Areas of Evaluation

King recommends that assessment of suitable candidates for sensori-motor-integrative treatment approaches include 1) observation, 2) person-drawing, 3) visual skills assessments, 4) auditory skills assessments, 5) tests of the central nervous system integration, 6) time relationships, 7) historical data, and 8) psychiatric history and status.[3]

Although not primarily intended for geriatric clients, the Comprehensive Evaluation of Basic Living Skills (CEBLS) is an excellent tool for clients in a community oriented program. This instrument involves assessments in personal care and hygiene; practical evaluation (meal planning, telephone, bus, shopping, meal preparation, serving and eating, and clean-up); written evaluation of reading, writing, and math skills; money transactions (counting, changing, budgeting, and banking); and time concepts. Copies of this evaluation can be obtained by writing:

> Jean Casanova
> 2185 North Hi Mount Boulevard
> Milwaukee, Wisconsin 53208

The Paracheck Geriatric Rating Scale is accompanied by a treatment manual (written in cooperation with Lorna Jean King). This validated and standardized (150 geriatric patients at Arizona State Hospital) assesment tool consists of three important categories: physical capabilities (ambulation, eyesight, and hearing), self-care skills (toilet habits, eating, hygiene, grooming), and social interaction skills (ward-work, individual responses, group activities). After the test is scored, the accompanying treatment manual provides specific treatment procedures and suggestions that are appropriate for each of the three treatment groups. The Paracheck Geriatric Rating Scale, Treatment Manual (in cooperation with L.J. King), and cumulative progress records are available from:

Greenroom Publications
8512 East Virginia Rd.
Scottsdale, Arizona 85257

Numerous evaluations and testing procedures in physical dysfunction are discussed in *Occupational Therapy Management of Physical Dysfunction.*[4]

The Home Health Service Occupational Therapy Evaluation and Care Plan (also known as the Occupational Therapy Evaluation and Care Plan) was developed by Ruth Levine, Lynn Marcus, Jane Roda, and Carmella Strano of the Community Occupational Therapy Consultants Group. The Evaluation and Care Plan evaluates the patient's home situation, physical capacity, and activities of daily living. It also provides for comments concerning treatment procedures, goals (both short and long term), and suggestions. The Evaluation can be found in *Willard and Spackman's Occupational Therapy* (fifth edition, 1978) and is available from J.B. Lippincott Company.

Other Evaluations

Five evaluations follow after a brief description of each:

The *Geriatric Occupational Therapy Assessment of Task Performance* by Laura Stravinskas utilizes a craft approach to assess motor, cognitive, psychological, social, and sensory-motor functioning.

The *Geriatric Assessment* by Elizabeth Murphy evaluates orientation, activities of daily living, motor skills, response to environment, communication skills, and a variety of other perceptions and skills (eg, differentiating geometric shapes and self-concepts by means of a self-drawing or recognizing one's self in mirror).

The *Geriatric Basic Status Form* by Sandra Lewis (primarily intended for the bed-confined older person) evaluates orientation, performance of simple cognitive activities, and response to sensory stimulation (tactile, olfactory, light pressure, deep pressure, and visual).

The *Geriatric Sensory Evaluation* by Laura Stravinskas and Sandra Lewis assesses the client's sensory functioning and general orientation status. This form is primarily designed for ambulatory clients involved in sensory training or sensory stimulation programs.

The *General Awareness Assessment* was written by Jeanette Liddle when she worked in the geriatric section of a large psychiatric hospital. During that time, it was difficult to procure appropriate evaluations for the older psychiatrically and physically impaired patient. Although the COTA's scope of responsibilities does not include evaluations, this assessment answered that need. The assessment evaluates awareness of the self and environment, fine motor coordination, gross motor skills, wheelchair activities, and grooming and toileting skills.

GERIATRIC OCCUPATIONAL THERAPY
ASSESSMENT OF TASK PERFORMANCE*

Part 1

NAME: _____

MALE   DATE: _____

FEMALE   BUILDING/WARD: _____

HANDDOMINANCE   R   L

I. **Materials:**

  A) 8" x 8" piece of wood, heavy cardboard, or posterboard.
  B) Box of tiles—assorted colors, sizes, shades.
  C) Glue
  D) Provide sample tile trivet: light against dark of any hue.

SAMPLE: 8" x 8"

By permission of Laura Stravinskas, OTR, Norristown State Hospital, Norristown, Pa.

II. **Procedure:**

A) Ask patient/client hand dominance, age, name, date, building.
B) Evaluator sits on patient/client's dominant side approximately two feet away.
C) Place box of tiles in position to encourage midline crossing (reaching should occur).
D) Sample trivet presented.
E) Evaluator explains to client:

> *This is an evaluation to help us see which group might be best for you. I will be writing some things to help me know you better.*

> *This is a glued tile trivet, I want you to make one just like this. Here is your piece of cardboard, tiles, and glue. Choose the tiles which will make the design the same and glue them in place.*

(Directions may be adapted, if patient/client has difficulty understanding.)

Evaluation of Performance

Part 2

COMPONENTS	COMMENTS
I. **Motor Component**	

I. **Motor Component**
  A) *Postural/Locomotion*
    1) Reaching
    2) Sitting
    3) Walking (observable on ward)

  B) *Prehension/Manipulation*
    1) Grasp
      a. Gross
      b. Fine
    2) Coordinated Finger Use
    3) Thumb and Fingers
    4) One hand holds—One hand manipulates

II. **Cognitive Component**
  A) *Communication*
    1) Verbal
    2) Nonverbal

  B) *Problem-Solving*
    1) Ability to group and classify

according to color and size.
2) Appropriate application of tiles to board.

C) *Directions*
   1) Ability to understand and act on verbal instructions.
   2) Memory Retention

D) *Time Management* (organization and efficiency)

E) *Relationship of Objects*
   1) To Self
   2) To Other Objects

F) *Perception*
   1) Spatial
   2) Form

III. **Psychological Components**
   A) *Reaction to Activity*
      1) Frustration
      2) Anxiety
      3) Fear
      4) Pride/Self-Confidence
      5) Other:

IV. **Social Component**
   A) *Relationship to Authority Figure* (Evaluation)
      1) Acceptant
      2) Hostile
      3) Other

   B) *Interaction*
      1) None
      2) Minimal
      3) Excessive
      4) Other

V. **Sensory-Motor Component**
   A) *Ability to Motor Plan*
      1) Gross
      2) Fine

   B) *Crossing Midline*

   C) *Perceptions*
      1) Figure-Ground

VI. **Other**

GERIATRIC ASSESSMENT†

CLIENT'S NAME _____   EVALUATOR _____

DATE _____

	yes	no	yes	no
I. Orientation				
A. *Time*				
Does the person know:				
day				
month				
year				
time of day				
B. *Place*				
Does the person know:				
where she/he is				
room number				
hall/ward/wing				
where she/he is now				
C. *Person*				
Does the person know:				
her/his name				
group leader's name				
person adjacent				
RN, LPN, Therapist, Dr				
Assts. in her/his area				

II. Activities of Daily Living

Can the person:
- wash self
- brush teeth
- comb hair
- feed self solids
- feed self liquids
- dress self
- control bladder
- know her/his way around

III. Motor Skills

Can the person:
- walk
- sit
- catch ball
- throw ball
- move to music
- grasp and release

IV. Response to Environment

Does person:
- respond to touch
- track an object
- respond to auditory
- respond to odor
- respond to taste
- respond with reflexes or repetitive movement
- imitate your movement

†*By permission of Elizabeth Murphy, OTR, Philadelphia, Pa.*

V. Communication

Can person:

mute

make self understood

speak on appropriate topic

initiate conversation

state a clear, logical sentence

respond to yes, no questions

VI. Miscellaneous

Can person:

draw picture of self

know difference of a square and circle

differentiate chair, bed, door, self

recognize self in mirror

If the person needs any assistance, check no.
If you wish to be more accurate please expand upon this and clarify the specific responses that you will expect (ie, *respond to auditory* means that the person will turn head in direction of a loud noise, or *know her way around* means knowing how to get from her room to specific places such as dining room, independently).

GERIATRIC BASIC STATUS FORM
OCCUPATIONAL THERAPY
NORRISTOWN STATE HOSPITAL*

CLIENT'S NAME _____

DATE _____

RECOGNITION:

	Idiosyncratic Identification	Is Able	Needs Assistance	Not Able
I. Orientation Status:				
Own name				
Name of one roommate				
Present location				
Season				
Date				
Own birthday				
Familiar song				

COMMENTS:

	Idiosyncratic Identification	Is Able	Needs Assistance	Not Able
II. Picture Identification:				
House				
Bird				
Dog				
Flower				
Holidays				

**By permission of Sandra Lewis, MFA, OTR, Norristown State Hospital, Norristown, Pa. July 1976.

COMMENTS:

III. **Tactile and Sensory Stimulation:**
    Smooth leather
    Rough leather
    Rough sandpaper
    Textured fabric
    Rough fabric
    Large mesh material
    Large plastic button
    Picture hook
    Empty spool of thread

COMMENTS:

IV. **Olfactory Stimulation:**
    Orange extract
    Peppermint extract
    Anise extract
    Garlic

COMMENTS:

V. **Skin and Topical Stimulation**
    A. Response to light pressure

COMMENTS:

    B. Response to massage:

        Skin appears:

GERIATRIC SENSORY EVALUATION‡

COMMENTS

I. Orientation
A. *Person:*
   1. What is your name? _____

   2. How old are you? _____

B. *Time:*
   1. What month is this? _____

   2. What is the date? _____

   3. What day of the week is it?__

   4. Is it morning or afternoon? _

   5. What is the season of the year? _____

C. *Place:*
   1. Where do you live?
      Ward/floor/building#/hospital

II. Sensory Components:
A. *Laterality & Directionality*
   (pencil)
   1. Take this with your right hand

   2. Take this with your left hand

   3. Move your arms up _____ ,
      down _____ , right side _____ ,
      left side _____

B. *Proprioception:* (1 and 3 lb.
   weights)
   1. (Place weights in patients
      hands)
      Which one is heavier? _____

‡*By permission of Laura Stravinskas, BS, OT, OTR, and Sandra Lewis, MFA, OTR.* Geriatric Sensory Evaluation © 1978.

C. *Body Positioning:*

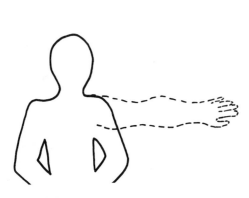

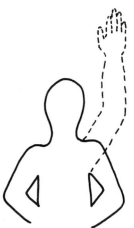

1. Trial (with vision)
Place patient's arm in the following position.* Ask patient
to assume same position with
other arm.

2. Repeat process with vision
occluded, using the following
position:

D. *Tactile:* (Duplicate objects, example: soft, hard, rough, fuzzy)
One set of objects is placed on
table in front of patient. Second
set is placed in closed box with
an opening for hands.
1. Patient is asked to touch an
object on table, then reach
into box and find it.

E. *Olfactory:*
a) Perfume/after shave saturated
paper
b) Garlic
1. How does this smell to you?
a. _____
b. _____

*Another position may be used.

F. *Gustatory:* (Jello)
   1. What does this taste like? (cold, hot, sweet, sour, lumpy, good, bad, smooth) _____
      _____

G. *Visual* (Distances, directionality, orientation status)
   1. Is this pen close (1′) or away (3′) from you?
      _____   _____

   2. Is this pen moving to the right or left (2′)?
      _____   _____

   3. Is this pen moving up or down? (2′)
      _____   _____

   4. Present 2 cubes of different sizes (example: 1″ and 3″ cubes)
      Which is the biggest of the 2 cubes?
      _____   _____

   5. Color identification cards (Present one card at a time)
      What color is this card?
      a. Red   b. Blue   c. Green

H. *Audition:* (Directionality, orientation status)
   Trial with vision (Ring bell approximately 3′ from patient)
   1. Point to the side you hear the sound coming from.
      Right _____   Left _____
   2. Repeat trial with vision occluded (left side first)
      Left _____   Right _____

General observations (anxiety, attention span, frustration levels....)
(Directions may be adapted to patients' functioning capacity)

NORRISTOWN STATE HOSPITAL
GERIATRIC OCCUPATIONAL THERAPY
GENERAL AWARENESS ASSESSMENT*

1) Independent — I
2) Supervision — S
3) Assistance — A
4) Not Able — N

COMMENTS

A. **Awareness of Environmental Factors**
    1) Name—
    2) Age—
    3) Place—
    4) Date—
    5) Names of Family—(Husband, Wife, Children)
    6) Names of two employees they have contact with—
    7) Name of one other patient—
    8) Location of:
        a. Dining Hall—
        b. Sleeping area—
        c. Bathroom—
        d. Water Fountains—

COMMENTS

B. **Description of Self**
    1) Hair Color
    2) Eye Color
    3) Skin Color
    4) Height
    5) Weight
    6) Draw a picture of self

*By permission of Jeanette Liddle, COTA, Norristown State Hospital, Norristown, Pa.

C. Fine Motor Coordination

1) Unilateral	Pick Up	Hold It	Manipulate in Hand	Place	Release
a. Orange Juice Can	___	___	___	___	___
b. Ball	___	___	___	___	___
c. Pencil	___	___	___	___	___
d. Coin	___	___	___	___	___
e. Pin	___	___	___	___	___
f. Self-Feeding Assessment	___	___	___	___	___
g. Handwriting—ask for signature					

2) Active Assistive
a. Paper in Envelope—
3) Simultaneous Activities
a. Clap Hands

COMMENTS

COMMENTS:
D. Grooming and Toileting Skills
1) Comb Hair
2) Brush Teeth
3) Wash Face
4) Dress Self
   a. Underwear
   b. Dress
   c. Socks
   d. Shoes

5) Toileting
   a. Sit on Commode
   b. Use Toilet Paper
   c. Flush Toilet
   d. Wash Hands

E. Gross Motor
1) Rising from Seat
2) Standing
3) Walking
   a. Forward Gait
   b. Walk on Line

COMMENTS

F. Wheelchair Activities
1) Propel:
   a. Forward
   b. Backward
   c. Turn
2) Transfer:
   a. Bed
   b. Chair
   c. Toilet

Summary and Additional Comments:

Treatment Plans

After the patient or client has been evaluated for his current functioning level, appropriate treatment should be planned and implemented (critical management); discussion and consensus with the professional team as to short term and long term goals and a prescription referral from the primary physician are essential.

Currently, the problem-oriented approach to documenting treatment is the method most often used by the majority of hospitals and agencies in the United States. This consists of identifying specific problem areas and administering appropriate treatment to alleviate and/or ameliorate the problem(s). For example, the appropriate occupational therapy intervention methods for an older client whose problem is shortness of breath can include graded exercise and activity, instruction in energy conservation principles and techniques, as well as work simplification, supplemental instruction in limitations, and family training and instruction.[5]

Progress Notes

Documentation of the patient's response to treatment is the

primary way accrediting agencies determine the quality of professional care giving. It is also a method for assessing the effectiveness of the treatment.

General Guidelines for Writing Progress Notes

1) Notes should be recorded every 30 days.

2) They must reflect the critical management (treatment) plan and show interaction with the patient.

3) Medicare and most other third party payers require the notes to show justification for continued treatment or hospitalization (unless the person is discharged) and demonstrate that the patient is receiving active treatment (not maintenance or custodial care).

4) Whenever there is a recommendation for a referral, there should be a referral form in the record (or an explanation as to why the action was not consummated).

5) Whenever occupational therapy services are discontinued, the reason must be recorded.

6) The date and name of service (department) should be indicated at the beginning of each note.

7) Occupational therapy progress notes should be signed at the bottom of the note with the therapist's full name and title.

8) If a student is writing the note it should be countersigned by the supervising therapist.

Staff Development

This discussion area speaks to the methods that are helpful in providing continuing professional growth and development.

1) Increased job responsibility.
2) In-Service and out-service education programs.
3) Rotation of assignments.
4) Attendance at professional meetings.
5) University courses, conferences, and field trips.
6) Study days.
7) Journal clubs.[6]

Doris C. Kaplan, OTR, director of a 27 person psychiatric occupational therapy department, discusses her experiences, thoughts, and feelings concerning staff development and related topics.

Interview with Doris Kaplan, OTR*

Lewis: How do you define staff development?

Kaplan: I think there are a number of parts. First, encourage people to grow professionally by providing them with opportunities for increased knowledge (in-service and out-service). Second, provide opportunities for increasing degrees of responsibility, and third, provide opportunities for feedback from peers and more experienced therapists.

Lewis: What have you found are the contributing factors that foster staff development?

Kaplan: I think the whole supervisory structure is a part of staff development.

Lewis: Why?

Kaplan: Because that is where people find out what they don't know and where the experienced leader (supervisor) provides modeling, shared leadership, and suggests resources to pursue for additional information.

Lewis: What can be done to keep staff aware of new programs and treatment methods?

Kaplan: The leadership of a department must be aware of professional developments both in one's field and allied fields.

I think one needs to read his/her own professional journals and publications, participate in his/her local professional organizations, and attend as many workshops and conferences as possible.

I'd like to go back to another aspect of staff development—that is, to provide an atmosphere in which people feel free to try new ideas. These ideas should be grounded in a good theoretical base, and there should be assurance that the outcome will not be damaging to the client.

Lewis: How do you develop leadership abilities among employees?

By permission of Doris Kaplan, O.T.R., Director of Occupational Therapy, The Norristown State Hospital, Norristown, Pa.

Kaplan: This is partly developed through clearly delineating the responsibilities of each position. It can also be accomplished by providing support and resources to carry them out. Other ways are to delegate responsibilities by developing a system for shared leadership—democratic participation in decision making, finding a way to say yes instead of no, and look for leadership potential in choosing staff, and then give these persons the opportunity to be leaders.

Lewis: How does one develop rapport and cooperation between different services and disciplines?

Kaplan: By a lot of hard work.

Lewis: Would you explain this?

Kaplan: One should participate in as many as possible of the appropriate multidisciplinary and interdepartmental activities, meetings, and committees as a willing and contributing member. Second, "selling" occupational therapy in terms of the mission of the institution/service/unit is of extreme importance. Finding out and using the informal power structure, and developing good interpersonal relationships at all levels, are other contributing factors.

Developing Community Information Exchange Projects

Not only do geriatric specialists have an obligation to organize professional educational experiences for fellow practitioners, they also should be committed to developing community educational opportunities for geriatric consumers.

There is a growing trend on the part of health care providers to be responsive to the consumer, and this is increasingly becoming an integral part of the total health care delivery concept. The consumer revolution demands that clients know more about treatment opportunities.

Therapist involvement in educationally-oriented community projects provides consumers and the community-at-large with information regarding occupational therapy skills and services.

As coordinator(s) of a geriatric community service and skill fair, occupational therapists have opportunities to come into contact with heads of agencies, numerous educational and health professionals, consumers, civic leaders, and the press. "The Highlights by Older Adults" program held at a shopping mall in Montgomery County, Pa, reflects this type of project. Sponsored by the Montgomery County Task Force on Older Adults (a voluntary citizen-consumer and professional organization interested in improving the quality of life of the older residents of the county), this organization selected an occupational therapist to be coordinator for their first effort (September, 1975).

Responsibilities for organizing this event included involving community service agencies to share information with consumers and developing a specific discussion and entertainment program. The goals for this project were to inform clients and citizens of existing human and health care services in the local community and to provide elders with an arena in which they can display their skills and achievements.

Because the budget was very limited (no more than $35.00 was available), all costs had to be kept to a minimum. The managerial methods involved establishing a locale that was cost-free and accessible to public transportation (a local shopping center) and contacting participating agencies and interested individuals by public service news media (cost-free news spots are allocated in most local newspapers if the project is nonprofit and open to the community), mail, telephone, and at group meetings.

Tables displaying hobby exhibits, art work, hand crafts, and agency information demonstrated the older person's skills and served to inform consumers of the types of services that are available to them in their local community. The agencies, organizations, and groups that exhibited included homemaker's home health aids, a bank (specialized services for older persons), nutrition programs, visiting nurse associations, nursing homes, a private craft group that only sells merchandise made by elders, numerous senior adult activities centers, retired senior volunteer program, a private employment agency that primarily councils older persons for possible employment opportunities, the County Geriatric and Rehabilitation Center, the County Public Library (featuring home bound services), the County Department of Consumer Affairs, and the Occupational Therapy Department at the nearby State Hospital.

The entertainment and discussion portion of this project featured the three County Commissioners (local governing body), the director for the County Area on Aging Agency, a panel of three elderly Retired Senior Volunteer Program participants, the Syncopated Seniors (a band composed of older persons who had earlier represented the United States as goodwill ambassadors to Romania), and a speaker from the Gray Panthers.

There were 20 exhibits and a total of 370 persons. This type of program created an awareness on the part of the community that agencies working cooperatively can produce a minimum cost program that involves consumers and providers.[7] It also provides a significant opportunity to become knowledgeable about occupational therapy offerings.

11

Challenges for the Future— Developing A Positive Therapeutic Model

Occupational therapists are challenged as never before to provide elders with substantive, therapeutic programs that improve the older person's ability to function independently as long as possible.

Some researchers believe that babies born within the next 35 years will have an opportunity to achieve a life expectancy of over 125 years. These same investigators also feel confident that by the year 2100 it will be possible to attain a life expectancy of 600 to 1,000 years.* These startling revelations make one realize that the therapist's obligations to older citizens will continue to flourish and magnify.

Myths About Aging

In Chapter 1 we had discussed ageism and explored some of the reasons for it. In reference to this concept, let us now examine some stereotypes and myths that are associated with older persons.

1. *Old People Are Unproductive.* Ninety-five percent of our older citizens live in their communities. One third of their total income comes from their own efforts. Another 45% is derived from pensions that they have earned through hard work during their full employment years. Still another 15% comes from their own savings. Surprisingly, only 5% of their income is derived from public assistance programs.[1] There are many older people who were creative in youth and who continued to be creative in

---

Living to age 1,000. The Philadelphia Evening Bulletin, *June 6, 1977, p 1.*

late years—some of these notables include the following:

Benjamin Franklin (1706-1790) was 70 when he helped to produce the Declaration of Independence, and at age 77 helped to negotiate the peace treaty that signalled the close of the American Revolution. At 80 years of age Franklin attended the Convention that drew up the Constitution.[1]

Imogen Cunningham (1883-1976) began taking pictures in 1901 and continued her photographic craft until her death at age 93.

Arthur Rubenstein's musical genius spans the decades. *Marc Chagall*, in his ninetieth year, continues to astonish the world with his poetic and brilliant art work.

2. *Old People Are Inflexible.* Studies demonstrate that the ability to adapt to changing situations has more to do with life-long character traits than with inherent aging.

3. *Older People Wish To Be Separated From The Mainstream.* While some older persons may choose to live alone or with others their own age, many would prefer to maintain themselves in familiar neighborhood surroundings. However, due to friends and family members who move away or die, they find they can no longer afford to live in their own homes. Instead, out of necessity, they often withdraw to live in age-segregated groups.

4. *Older Folks Are Content.* Many of our communication media show the carefree, cookie-baking grandmother or the benign, rocking-chair grandfather as a stereotype of old age. The facts are that a good many older people experience the devastating stresses and losses of aging. On the other hand, a number of researchers now believe that some stress is essential to living, and that older people who are totally protected from everyday stresses deteriorate at a rapid rate.[2]

Elders Changing the Image

So with age is wisdom and with length of days understanding. (Job 12:12)

From the discussion in the previous section, one could assume that older persons have become locked into a system that negates their existence as viable and productive human beings. However, elders are on the move to change this image. A recent article in the business section of the *New York Times* points out that as companies are facing more economic and marketing uncertainties, they are taking a closer look at the older, more seasoned executive. Some of these illustrious economic and business advisors are William M. Batten, former chairman of the J.C. Penney Company, who was called out of retirement at age 67 to become Chairman of the New York Stock Exchange, and William M. Blackie, a 72-year-old retired executive of Genesco, Inc., who was similarly called back to run the troubled company until its search committee was able to find a permanent chief executive. It is interesting to note that the committee chose John L. Hanigan, a 65-year-old former chief executive of the Brunswick Corporation, to head Genesco. The National Center for Career Life Planning of the American Management Associations (founded in October of 1975) was established to encourage companies, agencies, and organizations to utilize the experiences and talents of capable, older Americans. Two panels of leading citizens from a cross section of society have already been appointed to develop strategy, and seminars are scheduled to begin in the immediate future.†

R.N. Butler documents a number of changes that characterize the older person. Several of these including the *change in the sense of time* (emphasis on the quality of the present time), *sense of the life cycle* (accumulation of factual knowledge and a sense of the life experience), the *desire to leave a legacy,* and the *transmissions of power,* can be helpful factors in promoting a society that utilizes the skills and abilities of citizens who have, through the years, acquired a storehouse of information grounded in practical application.[3]

Perhaps the wise words of the founding fathers, written in Congress on July 4, 1776 as part of the Declaration of Independence, sums up best the justification for people of all ages seeking satisfying life experiences.

> We hold these truths to be self-evident, that all men are created equal, that they are endowed by their Creator with certain unalienable Rights, that among these are Life, Liberty, and the pursuit of Happiness.

†*Barmash I: New jobs for old hands.* The New York Times, *Section 3, May 29, 1977, pp 1, 7.*

Stereotypes Concerning Occupational Therapy

Unfortunately, a few occupational therapists have created an unpleasant public image of the profession. One of the most noticeable accountings of this can be found in a collection of word portraits based on the true-to-life reflections and experiences of older people—*Green Winter: Celebrations of Old Age.* One poem entitled "Occupational Therapy" speaks on this issue:

Preserve me from the occupational therapist, God,
She means well, but I'm too busy to make baskets.
I want to relive a day in July
When Sam and I went berrying
I was eighteen,
My hair was long and thick....
Oh, here she comes, the therapist, with scissors and paste.
Would I like to try decoupage?
"No," I say, "I haven't got time."
"Nonsense," she says, "you're going to live a long, long time."
That's not what I mean,
I mean that all my life I've been doing things
For people, with people, I have to catch up
On my thinking and feeling ...
"Please open your eyes," the therapist says,
"You don't want to sleep the day away."
As I say, she means well,
She wants to know What I used to do,
Knit? Crochet?
Yes, I did all those things,
and cooked and cleaned
and raised five children,
and had things happen to me.
Beautiful things, terrible things,
I need to think about them,
At the time there wasn't time,
I need to sort them out,
Arrange them on the shelves of my mind...[4]

It is clear that the therapist involved was only motivated to meet her own needs (ie, get the patient to make something). Thus, she overlooked her client's needs—to be permitted to openly participate in the life review process. Understanding the client's goals is the first priority in any therapeutic setting.

The Promise of Tomorrow

An occupational therapy program is much more than busy work; it consists of activities tailor-made to treat the specific condition of the client. Undertakings that provide satisfaction to elderly persons usually are related to experiences of their earlier years. Although old age brings changes in work, play, and family, the need for the satisfactions they provided remains ... Through evaluation of the client's current physical and psychological state and inquiry into satisfying experiences of previous years—especially the transition years between work and retirement—the occupational therapist plans a setting in which the person can best function. Through the treatment program, the occupational therapist strives to limit disability and reduce symptoms of physical or mental illness. In addition to its rehabilitative aspects, occupational therapy also prevents physical and mental deterioration through active and absorbing projects, group participation, and problem solving. Once the client's situation has been evaluated, the occupational therapist arranges for appropriate craft, homemaking, self-care, social, community, and interpersonal activities[5]

This description of occupational therapy services is a comprehensive view of the profession's goals and methods. There is much that we are doing, and with the dawning of advanced scientific inquiry and technology there will be more that we can do. Our quest for serving the older person can be summed up in this manner—without enthusiasm, compassion, love, and respect for the human spirit we cannot succeed; with treatment programs rooted firmly upon a knowledge base of current geriatric developmental and therapeutic theory, we cannot fail.

References

Chapter I

1. Butler RN, Lewis MI: Aging and Mental Health: Positive Psychosocial Approaches. Saint Louis, The CV Mosby Co, 1973, p 9.
2. Shakespeare W: As you like it. *In* Craig WJ (ed): The Complete Works of Shakespeare. New York, Oxford Univ Press, 1919, p 261.
3. Curtin S: Nobody Ever Died of Old Age. Boston, Little Brown & Co, 1973, p 3.
4. Albee E: Three Plays. New York, Coward-McCann Inc, 1960, pp 149, 150, 152, 1960.
5. Butler RN: An interview with Robert Butler. APA Monitor, March, 1976, pp 14-15.
6. Jones NA: Occupational therapy and the aged. Am J Occup Ther 28:615-618, 1974.
7. Goldfarb A, Frazier S: Aging and Organic Brain Syndrome. Fort Washington, Pa, McNeil Laboratories, 1974, p 5.

Chapter II

1. Rosen H et al: Working with Older People: A Guide to Practice. Washington, DC, Public Health Service Publications 1966, vol 1, no 1459, glossary.
2. Guilford JP: The Nature of Human Intelligence. New York, McGraw-Hill Book Co, 1967, p 24.
3. Biehler FR: Psychology Applied to Teaching. New York, Houghton Mifflin Co, 1971, p 78, 317-320.
4. Maier HW: Three Theories of Child Development. New York, Harper & Row Pubs Inc, 1969, pp 103-150.
5. Erikson EH: Childhood and Society. New York, WW Norton & Co Inc, 1963, pp 247-273.
6. Kohlberg L: Stages and aging in moral development—some speculations. The Gerontologist 1:497-502, 1973.
7. Cumming E, Henry WE: Growing Old: The Process of Disengagement. New York, Basic Books Inc, 1961, p 15.
8. Lidz T: The Person: His Development Throughout the Life Cycle. New York, Basic Books Inc, 1968, pp 483-484.
9. Neugarten B, Havighurst R, Tobin SS: Personality and patterns of aging. *In* Neugarten B (ed): Middle Age and Aging: A Reader in Social Psychology. Chicago, Univ Chicago Press, 1973, p 177.

Chapter III

1. Hall DA: The Aging of Connective Tissue. New York, Academic Press Inc, 1976, pp 3-4.
2. Busse EW: Theories of aging. *In* Busse EW, Pfeiffer E (eds): Behavior and Adaptation in Late Life. Boston, Little Brown & Co, 1969, pp 12-25.
3. Butler RN, Lewis MI: Aging and Mental Health: Positive Psychosocial Approaches. Saint Louis, CV Mosby Co, 1973, pp 102, 272-273.
4. Rosen H: Working with Older People: A Guide to Practice. Washington DC, Public Health Service Publication, 1966, vol 1, no 1459, p 13-17.
5. Hasselkus BR: Aging and the human nervous system. Am J Occup Ther 28:17-18, 1974.
6. Liang DS: Facts About Aging. Springfield, Illinois, Charles C Thomas Pubs, 1973, pp 8-11, 35, 36, 43.
7. Battle D: A speech therapist considers speech and hearing problems for the elderly. *In* Deichman ES, O'Kane CP (eds): Working with the Elderly: A Training Manual. Buffalo, New York, DOK Pubs Inc, 1975, pp 51-53.
8. Shore H: Designing a training program for understanding sensory losses in aging. Gerontologist 16:157-165, 1976.

Chapter IV

1. Ingraham MH: My Purpose Holds: Reactions and Experiences in Retirement of TIAA-CREF Annuitants. New York, Teachers Insurance and Annuity Association, 1974, p 59.
2. Barron ML: The Aging American: An Introduction to Social Gerontology and Geriatrics. New York, Thomas Y Crowell Co, 1961, p 78, 189.
3. Blau ZS: Old Age in a Changing Society. New York, Franklin Watts Inc, 1973, p 12, 138.
4. Medvedev ZA: Caucasus and Altay longevity: a biological or social problem? The Gerontologist 14:381-387, 1974.
5. Butler RN, Lewis M: Aging and Mental Health: Positive Psychosocial Approaches. Saint Louis, CV Mosby Co, 1973, pp 29-30.
6. Smith BK: Aging in America. Boston, Beacon Press Inc, 1973, pp 199-217.

Chapter V

1. Butler RN, Lewis M: Aging and Mental Health: Positive Psychosocial Approaches. Saint Louis, CV Mosby Co, 1973, pp 34, 50-60, 69, 74-80.
2. Butler RN: The life review: an interpretation of reminiscence in the aged. *In* Kastenbaum R (ed): New Thoughts on Old Age. New York, Springer Pub Co Inc, 1964, p 274.
3. Kastenbaum R, Aisenberg R: The Psychology of Death. New York, The Springer Pub Co Inc, 1972, p 252.
4. Beck AT: The Diagnosis and Management of Depression. Philadelphia, Pa, Univ Penn Press, 1973, pp 4-7.
5. Levin S: Depression in the aged: the importance of external factors. *In*

Kastenbaum (ed): New Thoughts on Old Age. New York, Springer Pub Co Inc, 1964, pp 179-188.

6. Goldfarb AI, Frazier S: Aging and Organic Brain Syndrome. Fort Washington, Pa, McNeil Laboratories Inc, 1974, pp 6-7.

7. Barbeau A: Long term assessment of levodopa therapy in Parkinson's disease. Can Med Assoc J 112:1379-1380, 1975.

8. Davis JC: Team management of Parkinson's disease. J Am Occup Ther 31:300-303, 1977.

9. Rodman GP, McEwen CG, and Wallace SL: Primer on the Rheumatic Diseases. New York, The Arthritis Foundation, 1973, pp 25-31, 78, 80-82.

10. Crain DC: The Arthritis Handbook: A Patient's Manual on Arthritis, Rheumatism, and Gout. New York, Exposition Press, 1972, pp 15-27, 31, 80, 109-121.

11. Rosen H et al: Working With Older People: A Guide to Practice. Washington DC, no 1459, vol 1, August 1966, p 14.

12. DeBakey ME et al: The President's Commission on Heart Disease, Cancer and Stroke: Report to the President. Washington DC, US Government Printing Office, vol 2. February 1965, pp 1, 14-162, 459.

13. Schnell HM, Jenkins JJ: Reduction of vocabulary in aphasia. In Sarno MT (ed): Aphasia: Selected Readings. Englewood Cliffs, New Jersey, Prentice-Hall Inc, 1972, pp 5, 17.

14. Battle D: A speech therapist considers speech and hearing problems for the elderly. In Deichman ES, O'Kane CP: Working with the Elderly: A Training Manual. Buffalo, New York, 1975, pp 57-58.

15. Dubos R, Maya P: Health and Disease. New York Time-Life Inc, 1965, p 96.

16. Laufer IJ, Kadison H: Diabetes Explained: A Layman's Guide. New York, Saturday Review Press, 1976, pp 35, 72, 97.

17. Trotter RJ (ed): Human insulin: Seizing the golden plasmid. Science News 114:195-196, September 16, 1978.

18. Beardwood JT Jr, Kelly H: Simplified Diabetic Management. Philadelphia, JB Lippincott Co, 1954, pp 4, 109-110, 113.

19. Danowski TS: Diabetes is a Way of Life. New York, Coward-McCann Inc, 1964, p 77.

Chapter VI

1. Barns EK, Sack A, Shore H: Guidelines to treatment approaches: modalities and methods for use with the aged. Gerontologist 13:515-518, 520, 1974.

2. Nursing Service, Guide for Reality Orientation. VA Hospital, rev ed. Tuscaloosa, Alabama, Feb 1970, pp 8-12.

3. Butler RN: The life review: an interpretation of reminiscence in the aged. In Kastenbaum R (ed): New Thoughts on Old Age. New York, Springer Pub Co Inc, 1964, p 266.

4. Butler RN, Lewis MI: Aging and Mental Health: Positive Psychosocial Approaches. Saint Louis, CV Mosby Co, 1973, pp 43-44.

5. Stonecypher DD Jr: Getting Older and Staying Young. New York, WW Norton Co Inc, 1974, pp 207-208, 211.

6. Webb LJ, Urner S, McDaniels J: Physiological characteristics of a champion runner. J Gerontol 33:286-290, 1977.

7. Leslie DK, McLure JW: Exercises for the Elderly. Des Moines, Iowa, Univ Iowa, 1973, pp 7-110.
8. Exercise and your heart. Consumer Reports. May 1977, p 256.
9. Frekany GA, Leslie DK: Effects of an exercise program on selected flexibility measurements of senior citizens. Gerontologist 15:182-183, 1975.
10. Stamford BA, Fallica A, Hambacker W: Effects of daily physical exercise on the psychiatric state of institutionalized geriatric mental patients. Res Q Am Assoc Health Phys Ed 45:34-41, 1974.
11. Fields S: Sage can be a spice in life. Innovations 4:11-18, 1977.
12. How to do range of motion of the arm and Hemipligic self ranging home exercise program. In Occupational Therapy for the Stroke Patient. Loma Linda, California, Loma Linda University Medical Center, August 20, 1974, pp 1-18.
13. Home exercises for the stroke patient: home exercise pulleys; and suggested relaxing exercises. In Occupational Therapy for the Stoke Patient. Loma Linda, California, Loma Linda University Medical Center, August 20, 1974, pp 19-22.
14. Davis JC: Team management of Parkinson's disease. Am J Occup Ther 26:300-308, 1977.
15. Principles of hand splinting. In Marshall E: Occupational Therapy Management of Physical Dysfunction. Loma Linda, California, Loma Linda University School of Allied Health Professions. August 1972, pp 118-123.
16. MacDonald EM: Occupational Therapy in Rehabilitation. Baltimore, Maryland, William S Wilkins Co, 1976, pp 166-171.
17. Hollis I: Rehabilitation of the Hand: a Two Day Seminar. Sponsored by the Delaware Occupational Therapy Association, Wilmington, Delaware, May 21-22, 1977.
18. Exercises for the patient: therapist exercises. In Marshall E: Occupational Therapy Management of Physical Dysfunction. Loma Linda, California, Loma Linda University, School of Allied Health Professions, August 1972, pp 86-87.
19. Hollis I: Splint substitutes. Am J Occup Ther 21:139-145, 1967.
20. Rossky EG: Protection of Arthritic Joints. Philadelphia, Moss Rehabilitation Hospital, 1976, pp 2-11.
21. Melvin JL: Rheumatic Disease: Occupational Therapy and Rehabilitation. Philadelphia, FA Davis Co, 1977.
22. Shore H: Designing a training program for understanding sensory losses in aging. Gerontologist 16:159-161, 1976.
23. Battle D: A speech therapist considers speech and hearing problems for the elderly. In Deichman ES, O'Kane CP (eds): Working with the Elderly: A Training Manual. Buffalo, New York, DOK Pubs Inc, 1975, pp 51-58.
24. Richman L: Sensory training for geriatric patients. Am J Occup Ther 23:254-257, 1969.
25. Ragsdale M: Montessori Motivational Toys Pamphlet. Doylestown, Pa, Montessori Educational Products, 1970.
26. Siev E, Freishat B: Perceptual Dysfunction in the Adult Stroke Patient: A Manual for Evaluation and Treatment. Thorofare, New Jersey, Charles B Slack Inc, 1976.
27. Dressing training for the stroke patient; putting on a short leg brace; putting on trousers; procedures for putting on and removing a cardigan with a dressing stick. In Occupational Therapy for the Stroke Patient. Loma Linda, California, University Medical Center, August 20, 1974, pp 24-39.
28. Lee MHM: Geriatric Medicine and Psychiatry: A Seminar. Sponsored by the

Norristown State Hospital, Norristown, Pa, February 6, 1976.

29. Lee MHM: Caring for the Elderly Patient at Home: A Family Guide (Activities of Daily Living). Nutley, New Jersey, Roche Laboratories, 1976.
30. Liang DS: Facts About Aging. Springfield, Illinois, Charles C Thomas Pubs, 1973, pp 23-27.
31. Kolodner EL: Neighborhood extension of activity therapy. Am J Occup Ther 27:381-383, 1973.
32. Matsutsuyu JS: The interest checklist. Am J Occup Ther 23:327, 1969.
33. Lewis S: A patient-determined approach to geriatric activity programming within a state hospital. Gerontologist 15:146-149, 1975.
34. King LJ: A sensory-integrative approach to schizophrenia. Am J Occup Ther 28:528-536, 1974.
35. Ayres AJ, Heskett WM: Sensory-integrative dysfunction in a young schizophrenic girl. J Autism Child Schizo 2:174-181, 1972.
36. Spelbring LM, Kirchman MM, Miller RB: The use of activities in rheumatic disease. Am J Occup Ther 19:260-261, 1965.

Chapter VII

1. Kastenbaum R, Aisenberg R: The Psychology of Death. New York, Springer Pub Co Inc, 1972, pp 191-193, 206-208, 218.
2. Knutson AL: Cultural beliefs on life and death. In Brim OG Jr et al: The Dying Patient. New York, The Russell Sage Foundation, 1970, pp 41, 43, 48.
3. Riley JW Jr: What people think about death. In Brim OG Jr et al: The Dying Patient. New York, The Russell Sage Foundation, 1970, pp 35-40.
4. Feifel H: Attitudes toward death in some normal and mentally ill populations. In Feifel H: The Meaning of Death. New York, McGraw-Hill Book Co, 1959, p 114.
5. Jeffers FC, Verwoerdt A: How the old face death. In Busse EW, Pfeiffer E: Behavior and Adaptation in Late Life. Boston, Little Brown & Co, 1969, p 171.
6. Kubler-Ross E: Questions and Answers on Death and Dying. New York, MacMillan Pub Co Inc, 1974, pp 1, 142-148.
7. Weisman AD: On Dying and Denying: A Psychiatric Study of Terminality. New York, Behavioral Pub Inc, 1972, pp 137, 145-150.
8. Levine S, Scotch NA: Dying: an emerging social problem. In Brim OG Jr et al: The Dying Patient. New York, The Russell Sage Foundation, 1970, p 218.
9. Sudnow D: Dying in a public hospital. In Brim OG Jr et al: The Dying Patient. New York, The Russell Sage Foundation, 1970, pp 192-195.
10. Lerner M: When, why and where people die. In Brim OG Jr et al: The Dying Patient. New York, The Russell Sage Foundation, 1970, pp 9, 21-22.
11. Fraser V, Thornton SM: The New Elders: Innovative Programs By, For and About the Elderly. Denver, Obenchain Printing Co, 1977, p 20.
12. Gammage SL, McMahon PS, Shanahan PM: The occupational therapist and terminal illness: learning to cope with death. Am J Occup Ther 30:294-299, 1976.

Chapter VIII

1. Isenhower RSW: Handbook on Third Party Reimbursement for Occupational

Therapy Services. Rockville, Maryland, American Occupational Therapy Association, October, 1976, Appendices A-5, pp 14, 19.
2. Porterfield JD: Perspectives on Accreditation. Chicago, Joint Commission on Accreditation of Hospitals, Nov-Dec 1976, p 1.
3. Bennett R, Eisdorfer C: The institutional environment and behavioral change. *In* Sherwood S (ed): Long-Term Care: A Handbook for Researchers, Planners and Providers. New York, Spectrum Pub Inc, 1975, p 392.
4. Butler RN, Lewis MI: Aging and Mental Health: Positive Psychosocial Approaches. Saint Louis, CV Mosby Co, 1973, pp 214-215.

Chapter IX

1. What Do You Want to be When You Grow Old? New York, Roerig-Pfizer, May 1976, ii.
2. Brody E: High risk groups among the elderly, their families and their communities. *In* Serving High Risk Groups Among the Elderly, Their Families and Their Communities. Madison, Wisconsin, Univ Wisconsin-Extension, Department of Social Work, 1972, pp 3-19.
3. Kiernat JM: Geriatric day hospital: a golden opportunity for therapists. Am J Occup Ther 30:285-288, 1976.
4. Aronson R: The role of the occupational therapist in a geriatric day hospital setting. Am J Occup Ther 30:290-292, 1976.
5. Williams R, Benes H: The day hospital at the Burke Rehabilitation Center. Am J Occup Ther 30:293, 1976.
6. Turbow SR: Geriatric group day care and its effect on independent living: a thirty-six month assessment. Gerontologist 15:508-510, 1975.
7. Menks F, Sittler S, Yanow B: A psychogeriatric activity group in a rural community. Am J Occup Ther 31:376-384, 1977.
8. Sherr VT, Eskridge OC, Lewis S: A mobile, mental-hospital-based team for geropsychiatric service in the community. J Am Geriatr Soc 24:363-365, 1976.
9. Hasselkus BR, Kiernat JM: Independent living for the elderly. Am J Occup Ther 27:181-188, 1973.

Chapter X

1. Bloom M: Evaluation instruments, tests and measurements in long-term care. *In* Sherwood S: Long-Term Care: A Handbook for Researchers, Planners and Providers. New York, Spectrum Pub Inc, 1975, pp 504, 575-577, 580, 583-584.
2. Lawton MP: Evaluation research in fluid systems. *In* O'Brien JE, Streib GF: Evaluative Research on Social Programs for the Elderly. Washington DC, Department of Health, Education and Welfare, 1977, p 9.
3. King LJ: Notes on Assessment (ᶜ 1975). Presented at a sensorimotor integrative treatment approach workshop at the Norristown State Hospital, Norristown, Pa, April 18-19, 1977.
4. Marshall E: Occupational Therapy Management of Physical Dysfunction. Loma Linda, California, Loma Linda University School of Allied Health Professions, August, 1972.

5. Kansas City Area Administrative Task Force: criteria for management of patients requiring occupational therapy. *In* Isenhower RSW: Handbook on Third Party Reimbursement for Occupational Therapy Services. Rockville, Maryland, American Occupational Therapy Association, October, 1976, pp A-23.
6. Occupational Therapy Manual on Administration. Dubuque, Iowa, WC Brown Pubs Co, 1968, p 23.
7. Lewis S: Community program unites OT and the consumer. Rockville, Maryland, OT Newsletter, July 1976.

Chapter XI

1. What Do You Want to be When You Grow Old? New York, Roering-Pfizer Pharmaceuticals, May 1976, p ii.
2. Growing Old: A Guide for Understanding and Help. Rockville, Maryland, American Occupational Therapy Foundation, Inc, 1976.
3. Butler RN: Why Survive? Being Old in America. New York, Harper & Row Pubs Inc, 1975, pp 409-418.
4. Maclay E: Green Winter: Celebrations of Old Age. New York, Reader's Digest Press, 1977, pp 46-48.
5. Terlizzi LP: Working with older people: occupations in therapy. Occup Outlook Quart (US Department of Labor, Bureau of Labor Statistics) Winter 1976, p 16.

Bibliography

Chapter II

Erikson EH: Identity and the life cycle: selected papers. Psychological Issues (Monograph). International Universities Press 1:1, 1959.

Ginsburg H, Opper S: Piaget's Theory of Intellectual Development. Englewood Cliffs, New Jersey, Prentice-Hall Inc, 1969.

Kohlberg L: Moral and religious education and the public schools: a developmental view. *In* Sizer R (ed): Religion and Public Education. Boston, Houghton Mifflin Co, 1967, pp 164-183.

Maslow AH: Toward a Psychology of Being, ed 2. Princeton, New Jersey, Van Nostrand Co, 1968.

Piaget J: The Psychology of Intelligence. London, Routledge and Kegan Paul, 1950.

Chapter III

Jennekins FGI, Tomlinson BE, Walton JN: Histochemical aspects of five limb muscles in old age. J Neural Sci 14:259-276, 1971.

Serratrice G, Roux H, Aquaron R: Proximal muscle weakness in elderly subjects. J Neural Sci 7:275-299, 1968.

Strehler BL: Time, Cells and Aging. New York, Academic Press Inc, 1962.

Chapter IV

Butler RN: Why Survive? Being Old In America. New York, Harper & Row Pubs Inc, 1975.

Friedmann EA, Havighurst RJ: The Meaning of Work and Retirement. Chicago, Univ Chicago Press, 1954, pp 1-9.

Harris L: The Myth and Reality of Aging in America. Washington, DC, National Council on the Aging Inc, 1975.

Toward a national policy on aging. White House Conference on Aging, vols 1, 2. Washington DC, Dept of Health, Education & Welfare, 1971.

Chapter VI

Boyes JH: Bunnell's Surgery of the Hand, ed 5. Philadelphia, JB Lippincott Co, 1970.

Clinical Symposium: Surgical Anatomy of the Hand. Summit, New Jersey, Ciba Pharmaceutical Products. vol 9, no 1, 1957.

Cowdry EV: The Care of the Geriatric Patient, (ed 2). Saint Louis, CV Mosby Co, 1963.

Hopkins HL, Smith HD (eds): Willard and Spackman's Occupational Therapy, ed 5.

Philadelphia, JB Lippincott Co, 1978.

Perry JA, Bevin AG: Evaluation procedures for patients with hand injuries. Phys Ther 54:593-598, 1974.

Wynn-Parry CB: Rehabilitation of the Hand, ed 3. London, Butterworths, 1973.

Chapter VII

Kubler-Ross E: On Death and Dying. New York, MacMillan Pub Co Inc, 1971.

Moore WE: Man, Time and Society. New York, John Wiley & Sons Inc, 1963.

Riley JW Jr: Death and bereavement. In International Encyclopedia of the Social Sciences. New York, Free Press, 1968.

Riley JW Jr: Old age in American society: notes on health, retirement and anticipation of death. J Am Soc Chartered Life Underwriters 22:27-32, 1968.

Chapter VIII

Activity Superviser's Guide. Washington DC, HEW—GPO#HSM73-6706. American Nursing Home Association. Contact: American Nursing Home Association, 1025 Connecticut Avenue NW, Washington, DC 20036.

Guidelines for Occupational Therapy Consultants to Long Term Care. Minneapolis, The Minnesota Occupational Therapy Association, 1975. Contact: Minneapolis Occupational Therapy Association, Box 822, Minneapolis, Minnesota 55440.

Planners and Instructors Guide. Rockville, Maryland, Division of Health Care Services. Contact: Office of Long Term Care, Division of Health Care Services, 5600 Fishers Lane, Rockville, Maryland 20852.

Restorative Occupational Therapy in the Extended Care Facility. Monrovia, California, 1971. Contact: Doris Kroulek, OTR, 6448 Don Julio Street, Long Beach, California 90815.

Stattely C, Goodman E, Lipson W (eds): The Occupational Therapist Consultant in Nursing Homes. New York, New York State Occupational Therapy Association, Metropolitan New York District. Contact: Cecilia Stattely, OTR, 189-45 45th Avenue, Flushing, New York, 11358.

Chapter IX

Brocklehurst JC: The Geriatric Day Hospital. London, King Edwards Hospital Fund, 1970.

Padula H: Developing Day Care for Older People, A Technical Assistance Manual. Washington DC, National Council on Aging Inc, 1972.

Preliminary Analysis of Select Geriatric Day Care Programs, Washington DC, Department of Health, Education and Welfare, Health Resources Administration, Bureau of Health Services Research, Division of Long-Term Care, 1974.

Chapter X

Lewis S: A geriatric program fair: the state hospital as an agent for community interaction. Hosp Community Psychiatry 27:154-159, 1976.

Index

A
Achlorohydria, 26
Adult day treatment centers, 122, 123
Ageism, 1
Aging, 7-29
  biological, 7, 19-29
  chronological, 7
  myths about, 159-160
  psychological, 7
  sociological, 7
  theories of aging and development, 7-16
Albee E, 3
American Association of Retired Persons, 34
Amyloidosis, 25
Aphasia, 55
Aphasic treatment programs, 84-85
Assessments
  Comprehensive Evaluation of Basic Living Skills, 137
  general view, 134-137
  Geriatric Assessment, 142-144
  Geriatric Basic Status Form, 145-146
  Geriatric Occupational Therapy Assessment of Task Performance, 139-141
  Geriatric Occupational Therapy General Awareness Assessment, 150-152
  Geriatric Sensory Evaluation, 147-149
  Home Health Services Occupational Therapy Evaluation and Care Plan, 138
  medical and clinical diagnostic measures, 45, 46
  Paracheck Geriatric Rating Scale, 137, 138
  Safe Exercising Pulse Test, 68, 69
Attitude therapy, 63, 64
Ayres LA, 94

B
Batten W, 161
Bender Visual-Motor Gestalt Test, 46
Biological changes, 19-29
  cardiovascular system, 25
  gastrointestinal tract, 26
  muscular system, 24
  nervous system, 24
  reproductive system, 25

respiratory system, 22
senses, 27-29
skeletal system, 23
skin and subcutaneous tissues, 26
urinary tract, 25, 26

Biological theories of aging, 20-22
accumulation of harmful materials, 20
accumulation of copying errors, 20
autoimmunity, 21
Curtis' Composite Theory, 21
decline in the doubling capacity of human cells, 20
DNA-RNA error, 21
eversion, 21
exhaustion, 20
genetic determinants of aging, 21, 22
index of cephalization, 21
intentional biological programming, 20
lipid peroxidation, 22
mean time failure, 20
stochastic theories, 21
Blackie W, 161
Bloom M, 135-136
Blue Cross, 39, 112
Brillman C, 116-120
Butler R, 4, 47, 161

C
Cancer, 56, 57
Carlson J, 75
Casanova J, 137
Cataracts, 28
Cerebral vascular accident, 55
Chagall M, 160
Changing roles, 33
Chronic health problem, 41
Climacteric, 25
Cochlea, 27, 28
Commission for Accreditation of Rehabilitation Facilities, 111
Community information exchange projects, 155-157
Community mental health care centers, 123-124
Community oriented programs, 121-122
Computerized axial tomogram, 45, 55
Consultancy, 109-120, 118
Consultant to activities leaders, 109, 110
Contracts, 113
Cunningham I, 160
Curtin S, 2
Craft modalities, 95-100

D
Day care, 121-122
Day hospitals, 122
Death, 101-107
  attitudes of professionals, 104
  comparative view, 101, 102
  dying process, 103
  factors affecting the coping process, 103
  hospice programs, 106
  places of death, 105, 106
  social death, 104, 105
  societal attitudes, 102, 103
Declaration of Independence, 161
Deleteriousness, 19
Decontextualization, 101
Direct service, 111
Diseases, 41-58
  arteriosclerotic psychosis, 47, 48
  cancer, 56, 57
  cerebral vascular accident, 55-56
  depression, 41-43
  depressive neuroses, 42
  diabetes mellitus, 58
  emphysema, 57
  gout, 52, 53
  heart disease, 53-55
  involutional meloncholia, 42
  manic depressive psychoses, 42
  neuroses, 44
  organic brain syndromes, 46, 47
  osteoarthritis, 50, 51
  osteoporosis, 23, 53
  paranoid states, 44
  parkinson's disease, 48, 49, 50
  personality disorders, 45
  presenile dementia, 48
  psychophysiological disorders, 45
  psychosomatic disorders, 45
  psychotic depressive reactions, 42
  rheumatoid arthritis, 51, 52
  senile psychosis, 47
  schzophrenia, 43
Documentation, 118, 134-137, 152, 153
Double simultaneous stimulations of the hand and face, 46

E
Emphysema, 57
Endorphins, 43
Enkephalins, 43

Erickson E, 8, 11-14
Evaluations; see assessments
Exercise
   arthritic exercise program, 78
   generalized group program, 68-72
   hemiplegic program, 72-74

F
Federal guidelines, 121
Federal Register, 39, 110
Federal regulations and standards, 109-111
Franklin B, 160
Friedman EA, 32
Freishat B, 85

G
Garfunkle A, 2
Glaucoma, 29
Goldfarb AI, 47
Gout, 52, 53
Gray Bears, 34
Gray Panthers, 34
Green Winter; Celebrations of Old Age, 162
Grodinsky L, 114-116

H
Hand management, 76-78
Hanigan JL, 161
Havighurst R, 16, 32
Heart disease, 53-55
   cardiovascular-renal disease, 54, 55
   cerebrovascular disease, 53
   diseases of the circulatory system, 54
Hemiplegia, 55
Hemiplegic rehabilitation nursing home program, 115, 116, 119, 120
Henry WE, 16
Hill L, 85
Hollis I, 77, 78
Home health care agencies, 126, 127
Hospice, 106
Housing needs, 33
Hypotonia, 24

I
Indirect service, 109
Industrial revolution, 2
Institutions, 33
Insulation, 101
Intrinsicality, 19

Interviews with
  Brillman C, 116-120
  Grodinsky L, 114-116
  Kaplan D, 154, 155
  Levine R, 128-130
  Parker SC, 130, 131
Involutional Melancholia, 42

J
Joint Commission on Accreditation of Hospitals, 111
Joints: positioning, protection, and energy conservation, 79, 80
Jones NA, 4

K
Kiernat JM, 121
King LJ, 93, 94, 137
Kohlberg L, 14, 15
Kolodner E, 91
Kubler-Ross E, 103, 104
Kyphoscoliosis, 23

L
Lawton MP, 136
Levine R, 128-130, 138
Lewis S, 138, 139, 142, 143, 147
Liddle J, 139, 150
Life Review, 67, 68
Life Skills Program
  cooking and menu planning, 88, 89
  grooming and dressing techniques, 86, 87
  self-feeding, 87
  transfer techniques, 87, 88
  work simplification, 90
Lidz T, 16
Lipofuscin, 25
Loss of
  auditory sense, 27, 28
  gustatory and olfactory senses, 29
  job, 32
  kinesthetic sense, 29
  life partner, 34
  physical capabilities, 31
  tactile sense, 29
  visual sense, 28
M
Manic depressive psychoses, 42
Marcus L, 138
Matsutsuyu JS, 91
Marshall E, 74

Maslow A, 15
Medicaid, 38
Medicare, 38, 118, 126, 127
Medullary olives, 24
Melvin JL, 80
Menopause, 25
Mental Status Evaluation, 46
Mental Status Questionnaire, 46
Model Cities Funding, 39
Murphy L, 138, 142-144

N

National Caucus for the Black Aged, 34
National Center for Career Life Planning, 161
National Institute of Aging, 37
National Institute of Mental Health, 37
Neighborhood center programs, 125, 126
Neighborbood Extension of Activity Therapy, 91
Neugarten B, 16
Neuroses
  hypochondriacal, 44
  hysterical, 44
  phobic, 44
  psychophysiological disorders, 45
  psychosomatic disorders, 45
Nursing homes
  extended care facilities, 112
  intermediate care facilities, 112
  proprietary, 112
  skilled nursing care facilities, 112

O

Occupational therapy program, 163
Older Americans Act, 35-37
  Title I — declaration of objectives, 35
  Title II — administration on aging, 35
  Title III — grants for state and community programs, 35
  Title IV — training and research, 35
  Title V — multipurpose senior centers, 36
  Title VI — national older Americans volunteer programs, 36
  Title VII — nutrition programs, 36
  Title VIII — amendments to other acts, 36
  Title IX — community service employment for older Americans, 36, 37
  Title X — middle-aged and older workers training act, 37
Opportunities for increased learning, 65, 66
Organic brain syndrome
  acute, 46
  chronic, 47
Organizing workshops and seminars, 133, 134

Osteoarthritis, 50, 51
Osteoporosis, 23, 53

P
Paranoid states, 44
Parker SC, 130, 131
Parkinson's disease, 48-50
Parkinsonian treatment team program, 75, 76
Periosteum, 53
Personality disorders, 45
Piaget J, 8, 9 10
Presbycusis, 28
Presbyopia, 28
Presenile dementia, 48
Private practice, 111, 114, 115, 118
Programs to prevent institutionalization, 124, 125
Progress notes, 152, 153
Progressiveness, 19
Psychosis
  arteriosclerotic, 47
  senile, 47
Psychotic depressive reactions, 42
Purkinje cells, 24

R
Reality orientation, 61-63
Reimbursement, 112
Relaxing techniques, 73, 74
Remotivation, 64, 65
Retirement
  mandatory, 2
  years, 31
Rheumatoid arthritis, 51, 52
Roda J, 138
Roosevelt FD, 31
Rossky E, 78
Rubenstein A, 160

S
Seborrheic keratoses, 26
Sexual activity, 25
Seminars, 133, 134
Senior action alliance centers, 34
Sensorimotor integration, 93-95
Sensorineural hearing loss, 27, 28
Schizophrenia, 43
Shakespeare W, 1
Short Portable Mental Status Questionnaire, 46
Siev E, 85

Simon P, 2
Social security, 31, 138, 121
Staff development 153-155
Strano C, 138
Stravinskas L, 138, 139, 147
Sudnow D, 105

T
Technology, 101
Theradoh, 78
Tobin SS, 16
Transposition, 101
Treatment plans, 152
Treatment programs
   adult day treatment centers, 122, 123
   aphasic patient programs, 84, 85
   arthritic exercise program, 78
   attitude therapy 63, 64
   avocational pursuits, 90-92
   client determined approaches, 92, 93
   community mental health care centers, 123-124
   cooking and menu planning, 88, 89
   development and training of sensory skills, 80-84
   day hospitals, 122
   grooming and dressing techniques, 86, 87
   generalized group exercise program, 68-72
   hemiplegic exercise program, 72-74
   hemiplegic rehabilitation nursing home program, 115, 116, 119, 120
   home health care agencies, 126, 127
   informational sources, 74, 75
   joint positioning, protection, and energy conservation, 79, 80
   life review, 67, 68
   neighborhood center programs, 125, 126
   neighborhood extension of activity therapy, 91
   nursing home responsibilities (occupational therapy services), 117
   opportunities for increased learning, 65, 66
   parkinsonian team management, 75, 76
   programs to prevent institutionalization, 124, 125
   reality orientation, 61-63
   relaxing techniques, 73-74
   remotivation, 64, 65
   role of the therapist, 61
   self-feeding, 87
   senior actualization and growth explorations, 71
   sensorimotor integration, 93-95
   therapeutic hand management, 76-78
   transfer techniques, 87, 88
   transitional residency program, 130, 131
   work simplification, 90

U
United Nations Demographic Year Book, 182
Universality, 19

W
White house conference on aging, 39
workshops, 133, 134